中国器官捐献和移植发展报告

（2023）

主　编　黄洁夫

清华大学出版社
北京

本书封面贴有清华大学出版社防伪标签，无标签者不得销售。

版权所有，侵权必究。举报：010-62782989，beiqinquan@tup.tsinghua.edu.cn。

图书在版编目（CIP）数据

中国器官捐献和移植发展报告 . 2023 / 黄洁夫主编 . -- 北京：清华大学出版社，2025.4.
ISBN 978-7-302-67942-4

Ⅰ . R193.3；R617

中国国家版本馆 CIP 数据核字第 20251VQ914 号

责任编辑：孙　宇
封面设计：钟　达
责任校对：李建庄
责任印制：刘　菲

出版发行：清华大学出版社
　　　　　网　　址：https://www.tup.com.cn，https://www.wqxuetang.com
　　　　　地　　址：北京清华大学学研大厦 A 座　　邮　　编：100084
　　　　　社 总 机：010-83470000　　邮　　购：010-62786544
　　　　　投稿与读者服务：010-62776969，c-service@tup.tsinghua.edu.cn
　　　　　质量反馈：010-62772015，zhiliang@tup.tsinghua.edu.cn
印 装 者：三河市君旺印务有限公司
经　　销：全国新华书店
开　　本：165mm×235mm　　印　张：15.75　　字　数：220 千字
版　　次：2025 年 4 月第 1 版　　印　次：2025 年 4 月第 1 次印刷
定　　价：98.00 元

产品编号：110374-01

《中国器官捐献和移植发展报告（2023）》
编委会

主　编：黄洁夫
主　审：高光明
副主编：高新强　赵洪涛　侯峰忠　郭建阳
　　　　郑树森　张　旭　叶啟发　王海波
　　　　陈静瑜　郑　哲
编　委：（以姓氏汉语拼音为序）
　　　　陈　峻　陈俊丽　陈莉萍　陈斯鹏
　　　　董　乾　杜　冰　范晓礼　胡春晓
　　　　黄　洁　黄　曼　黄　伟　金海龙
　　　　李　萌　林李艳　刘麟炜　刘　璐
　　　　刘　盛　苗慧波　慕　强　蒲　苗
　　　　史　赢　吴　波　熊天威　徐　骁
　　　　张天宇　周志强　周稚烨
译　者：赵　婕

Editorial Committee of the *Report on the Development of Organ Donation and Transplantation in China (2023)*

Editor-in-chief: Huang Jiefu

Chief reviewer: Gao Guangming

Deputy editor-in-chief: Gao Xinqiang, Zhao Hongtao
Hou Fengzhong, Guo Jianyang
Zheng Shusen, Zhang Xu, Ye Qifa
Wang Haibo, Chen Jingyu, Zheng Zhe

Editorial board: Chen Jun, Chen Junli, Chen Liping
Chen Sipeng, Dong Qian, Du Bing
Fan Xiaoli, Hu Chunxiao, Huang Jie
Huang Man, Huang Wei, Jin Hailong
Li Meng, Lin Liyan, Liu Linjiong, Liu Lu
Liu Sheng, Miao Huibo, Mu Qiang
Pu Miao, Shi Ying, Wu Bo, Xiong Tianwei
Xu Xiao, Zhang Tianyu, Zhou Zhiqiang
Zhou Zhiye

Translator: Zhao Jie

前　言

在国家卫生健康委、中国红十字会的指导支持下，由中国器官移植发展基金会组织编写的《中国器官捐献和移植发展报告（2023）》付梓。

自 2018 年 3 月第一部《中国器官移植发展报告》启动编写以来，时至今日已连续出版五部，成为中国器官捐献和移植官方权威数据来源。

中国政府高度重视发展人体器官捐献与移植事业，过去十多年，随着临床医学的进步及相关法规制度的完善，尤其是 2007 年 5 月起《人体器官移植条例》的施行，我国人体器官捐献和移植事业取得了长足进步。例如，2016 年，国家交通、航空、铁路等六部门联合建立了器官转运绿色通道，为拯救生命赢得了宝贵时间；2017 年 5 月，《中华人民共和国红十字会法》修订，明确要推动器官捐献工作，探索了慈善机构等开展人道主义救助机制；2021 年正式实施的《中华人民共和国民法典》中也明确了器官捐献的基本规则；2021 年 7 月由国家卫生健康委、国家发展改革委、财政部等七部委联合出台的《人体捐献器官获取收费和财务管理办法（试行）》明确人体器官获取使用成本，着力建立完善人体器官获取收费管理机制，有力推进器官移植法制化进程，是中国器官捐献移植改革的历史性进步。

2023 年 12 月《人体器官捐献和移植条例》的正式颁布标志着我国器官捐献和移植事业迈上了新台阶，进入了新的发展阶段。此次条例的修订，在名称中新增了"捐献"二字，这一变化凸显了器官捐献的重要性，也彰显了党和国家对于器官捐献移植事业的高度认可和推动这项大爱事业高质量发展的信心和决心。《中国器官移植发展报告》也从今年起正式更名为《中国器官捐献和移植发展报告》。至此，以捐献为前提的中国器官移植事业将在阳光下继往开来，砥砺前行。

习近平总书记在党的二十大报告中提出，推进健康中国建设，把保障人民健康放在优先发展的战略位置，完善人民健康促进政策。在世界卫生与健康领域，中国持续发挥着重要作用。同时，中国的卫生与健康事业也受益于国际间的相互支持。近年来，我国主动加强与各国的交流合作，全面展现了器官移植的顶层规划、制度构建、法律法规以及工作体系。通过世界卫生组织全球器官移植监测网，向国际社会公开提供相关数据及分析成果，以透明之态呈现我国人体器官捐献与移植工作的显著成效。

党的二十大强调增进民生福祉，提高人民生活品质。在新的时代背景下，新的时代赋予器官移植更高使命。我们将锲而不舍地奋进，构建一个完备且契合伦理规范、符合世界卫生组织准则的器官捐献与移植体系，全力攀登器官移植科学技术的新高峰。

本报告是中国器官移植发展基金会组织编写并连续出版的第五部报告，是中国器官移植发展改革成果的忠实记录。本次报告的出版，不仅是对过往工作的深度总结和提炼，更是对未来发展方向的清晰洞察和精准把握。在连续出版的历程中，我们不断积累经验、完善内容，而本次出版更是在前几部的基础上，融入了最新的研究成果、实践经验和国际前沿理念，为推动中国器官捐献和移植事业的发展提供了更具前瞻性和指导性的参考，也为全球器官移植领域贡献了独特的中国智慧和中国方案。中国器官移植发展基金会将继续秉承使命，以本报告为基石，为推动我国器官移植事业的蓬勃发展不懈努力。

《中国器官捐献和移植发展报告（2023）》编委会

2024 年 10 月

注：《中国器官捐献和移植发展报告（2023）》数据统计时间：2023 年 1 月 1 日—2023 年 12 月 31 日；数据统计范围为 31 个省（自治区、直辖市）及新疆生产建设兵团（不含中国香港特别行政区、澳门特别行政区和台湾省）。

Preface

Under the guidance and support of the National Health Commission and the Red Cross Society of China, the *Report on Organ Donation and Transplantation in China (2023)* organized and compiled by the China Organ Transplantation Development Foundation has been published.

Since the release of the inaugural *Report on Organ Transplantation in China* in March 2018, five volumes have been published consecutively, establishing itself as the official and authoritative source of data on organ donation and transplantation in China.

The Chinese government places great importance on the development of human organ donation and transplantation. Over the past decade, with the advancement of clinical medicine and the improvement of relevant laws and regulations, especially the implementation of the *Regulations on Human Organ Transplantation* since May 2007, significant progress on organ donation and transplantation has been made in China. For instance, in 2016, six ministries including transportation, aviation, and railway, etc., jointly issued the *Notice on the Establishment of a Green Channel for the Transport of Human Donor Organs*, thereby establishing the green channel for the swift transport of human donor organ in order to save time for life-saving activities; in May 2017, the *Law of the People's Republic of China on the Red Cross Society* clarified the responsibilities of the Red Cross Society of China in facilitating organ donation, and exploration on establishing the mechanism of humanitarian assistance by charitable organizations has started ever since; in 2021, the *Civil Code of the People's Republic of China* was taken into effect, clearly stipulating the basic rules of organ donation; in July 2021, the *Interim Provisions on Financial Management of Human Organ Procurement* jointly issued by seven ministries clarified the cost of organ procurement and utilization, with a focus on establishing and improving the financial management mechanism on issues regarding human organ procurement procedures. This has significantly accelerated the organ transplant legalization process, representing a landmark development in China's organ donation and transplant reform.

In December 2023, the official promulgation of *the Regulations on Human Organ Donation and Transplantation* marked a new milestone in China's organ donation and transplantation, ushering it into a new stage of development. One of the most significant revisions to *the Regulation* was the addition of Donation to the title, which highlighted the importance of organ donation and demonstrated the Chinese government's commitment to organ donation and transplantation, as well as its confidence and determination to advance this cause of great love. Consequently, from this year on, the *Report on Organ Transplantation Development in China* has also be officially renamed to the *Report on Organ Donation and Transplantation Development in China*. Henceforth, organ transplantation in China, which is founded on organ donation, will persist in its pursuit of advancement in the public eye.

This year marks the beginning of fully implementing the spirit of the 20th National Congress of the Communist Party of China. The report of the 20th National Congress presented by President XI Jinping stated that, (we must) *advance the Healthy China Initiative, give strategic priority to ensuring the people's health and improve policies on promoting public health.* China remains a significant player in the global health sector. Concurrently, China's health initiatives are also bolstered by international assistance. In recent years, China has taken the initiative to enhance exchanges and cooperation with a variety of countries, demonstrating the top-level planning, institutional construction, laws and regulations, and work systems of organ transplantation. At the same time, China provides relevant data and analysis results to the international community through the World Health Organization's Global Observatory on Donation and Transplantation, presenting the significant achievements of organ donation and transplantation related works in the country with transparency.

The 20th National Congress of the Communist Party of China emphasized the enhancement of people's well-being and the improvement of quality of life. Against the backdrop of the new era, organ transplantation has been endowed with a higher mission. We will persevere and strive to build a comprehensive organ donation and transplantation system that aligns with ethical standards and conforms to the guidelines provided by the World Health Organization, and make every effort to reach new heights in science and technology development of organ transplantation.

This report is the fifth edition compiled by the China Organ Transplantation Development Foundation, which is a faithful record of the achievements of reform on organ transplantation development in China. The publication of this report is not only an in-depth summary and refinement of past work but also a clear insight and precise grasp of directions for future development.

As a result of the ongoing publication process, We have acquired experience and enhanced the quality of content. This publication, based on the previous editions, incorporates the latest research findings, practical experience, and international cutting-edge concepts. It provides more forward-looking and guiding references for promoting the development organ donation and transplantation in China, and also contributes unique Chinese wisdom and solutions to the global field of organ transplantation. The China Organ Transplantation Development Foundation will continue to uphold its mission, taking this report as a cornerstone, and make unremitting efforts in promoting the vigorous development of organ transplantation in China.

Editorial Committee of the Report on the Development
of Organ Donation and Transplantation in China
October, 2024

NOTE: Time period for data collection of *Report on the Development of Organ Donation and Transplantationin China (2023)*: January 1, 2023 to December 31, 2023. Data of 31 provinces (autonomous regions and municipalities) and the Xinjiang Production and Construction Corps (excluding Hong Kong SAR, Macao SAR, and Taiwan Province) were included.

目 录

第一章 中国人体器官捐献 ························· 1
  一、机构和队伍建设情况 ························· 1
  二、志愿登记情况 ······························· 3
  三、器官捐献情况 ······························· 5
  四、相关工作开展 ······························· 7
  五、工作展望 ··································· 9

第二章 中国人体捐献器官获取 ····················· 10
  一、人体捐献器官获取体系建设与发展 ············· 11
  二、OPO 机构分布与建设情况 ···················· 12
  三、器官捐献情况 ······························· 13
  四、器官获取与利用情况 ························· 14
  五、捐献器官质量情况 ··························· 16
  六、特点与展望 ································· 18

第三章 中国人体器官分配与共享 ··················· 20
  一、中国移植医疗机构分布 ······················· 22
  二、人体器官捐献情况 ··························· 22
  三、移植等待者情况 ····························· 24
  四、人体器官分配与共享政策实施效果 ············· 28
  五、特点与展望 ································· 30

第四章 中国肝脏移植 ····························· 32
  一、肝脏移植医疗机构分布 ······················· 33

二、肝脏移植受体人口特征⋯⋯⋯⋯⋯⋯⋯⋯⋯⋯⋯⋯⋯⋯⋯⋯ 35

　　三、肝脏移植质量安全分析⋯⋯⋯⋯⋯⋯⋯⋯⋯⋯⋯⋯⋯⋯⋯⋯ 36

　　四、特点与展望⋯⋯⋯⋯⋯⋯⋯⋯⋯⋯⋯⋯⋯⋯⋯⋯⋯⋯⋯⋯ 39

第五章　中国肾脏移植⋯⋯⋯⋯⋯⋯⋯⋯⋯⋯⋯⋯⋯⋯⋯⋯⋯⋯⋯⋯ 41

　　一、肾脏移植医疗机构分布⋯⋯⋯⋯⋯⋯⋯⋯⋯⋯⋯⋯⋯⋯⋯⋯ 42

　　二、肾脏移植受体人口特征⋯⋯⋯⋯⋯⋯⋯⋯⋯⋯⋯⋯⋯⋯⋯⋯ 48

　　三、肾脏移植质量安全分析⋯⋯⋯⋯⋯⋯⋯⋯⋯⋯⋯⋯⋯⋯⋯⋯ 49

　　四、特点与展望⋯⋯⋯⋯⋯⋯⋯⋯⋯⋯⋯⋯⋯⋯⋯⋯⋯⋯⋯⋯ 51

第六章　中国心脏移植⋯⋯⋯⋯⋯⋯⋯⋯⋯⋯⋯⋯⋯⋯⋯⋯⋯⋯⋯⋯ 53

　　一、心脏移植医疗机构分布⋯⋯⋯⋯⋯⋯⋯⋯⋯⋯⋯⋯⋯⋯⋯⋯ 53

　　二、心脏移植受体人口特征⋯⋯⋯⋯⋯⋯⋯⋯⋯⋯⋯⋯⋯⋯⋯⋯ 56

　　三、心脏移植质量安全分析⋯⋯⋯⋯⋯⋯⋯⋯⋯⋯⋯⋯⋯⋯⋯⋯ 57

　　四、特点与展望⋯⋯⋯⋯⋯⋯⋯⋯⋯⋯⋯⋯⋯⋯⋯⋯⋯⋯⋯⋯ 59

第七章　中国肺脏移植⋯⋯⋯⋯⋯⋯⋯⋯⋯⋯⋯⋯⋯⋯⋯⋯⋯⋯⋯⋯ 61

　　一、肺脏移植医疗机构分布⋯⋯⋯⋯⋯⋯⋯⋯⋯⋯⋯⋯⋯⋯⋯⋯ 62

　　二、肺脏移植受体人口特征⋯⋯⋯⋯⋯⋯⋯⋯⋯⋯⋯⋯⋯⋯⋯⋯ 64

　　三、肺脏移植质量安全分析⋯⋯⋯⋯⋯⋯⋯⋯⋯⋯⋯⋯⋯⋯⋯⋯ 66

　　四、特点与展望⋯⋯⋯⋯⋯⋯⋯⋯⋯⋯⋯⋯⋯⋯⋯⋯⋯⋯⋯⋯ 70

第八章　中国器官移植技术进展与创新⋯⋯⋯⋯⋯⋯⋯⋯⋯⋯⋯⋯⋯⋯ 73

　　一、劈离式肝移植关键技术体系建立和推广⋯⋯⋯⋯⋯⋯⋯⋯⋯⋯ 73

　　二、甲胎蛋白－谷氨酰转肽酶－杭州标准评分（AFP-GGT-Hangzhou scoring system，AGH 评分）是肝细胞癌患者肝移植术后无病生存和靶向治疗效果的预测指标⋯⋯⋯⋯ 75

　　三、融合双分子标志物的肝癌肝移植患者分类新标准⋯⋯⋯⋯⋯⋯ 79

　　四、天然高分子生物肝材料治疗多器官功能衰竭核心技术体系的建立与应用⋯⋯⋯⋯⋯⋯⋯⋯⋯⋯⋯⋯⋯⋯⋯⋯⋯ 80

　　五、基于基因模型指导肝移植术后抗排异反应精准给药方案⋯⋯ 82

　　六、达芬奇机器人辅助腹腔镜技术在肾移植中的应用⋯⋯⋯⋯⋯⋯ 83

七、人工血管保护外鞘预防移植肾动脉扭折的疗效 …………… 86
八、六基因编辑猪-恒河猴异种肾脏移植 …………………………… 88
九、国内首组婴幼儿供肾给婴幼儿肾移植 37 例 ………………… 90
十、无缺血心脏移植 …………………………………………………… 91
十一、一种全新的心肌活检技术在心脏移植术后的应用 ………… 92
十二、基于机器学习的肺移植患者预后模型 ……………………… 94
十三、机器人辅助微创入路单肺移植手术 ………………………… 95
十四、供体来源游离 DNA 在肺移植术后排异反应
　　　诊断中的应用 ………………………………………………… 97

索　引 ………………………………………………………………… 99

Contents

Chapter 1   Human Organ Donation in China **101**
    1.1   Organizations and team building 102
    1.2   Registration of human organ donation volunteers 105
    1.3   Organ donation in China 107
    1.4   Progress of related work 109
    1.5   Future outlook 113

Chapter 2   Donated Organ Procurement in China **115**
    2.1   Development and construction of human donated organ procurement system 116
    2.2   Distribution and construction of OPOs 118
    2.3   Organ donation in China 119
    2.4   Procurement and utilization of organs 121
    2.5   Quality of donor organs 123
    2.6   Features and future outlook 125

Chapter 3   Human Organ Allocation and Sharing in China   129
    3.1   Distribution of transplant hospitals in China 132
    3.2   Overview of human organ donation 133
    3.3   Patients waiting for organ transplantation 135
    3.4   Policy implementation efficacy in organ allocation and sharing   140
    3.5   Feature and future outlook 142

Chapter 4   Liver Transplantation in China **145**
    4.1   Distribution of medical institutions qualified for liver transplantation 146
    4.2   Demographic characteristics of liver transplant recipients 149
    4.3   Quality and safety analysis of liver transplantation 150

  4.4 Feature and future outlook 153

Chapter 5 Kidney Transplantation in China 156
  5.1 Distribution of medical institutions qualified for kidney transplantation 157
  5.2 Demographic characteristics of kidney transplant recipients ... 165
  5.3 Quality and safety analysis of kidney transplantation 166
  5.4 Feature and future outlook 169

Chapter 6 Heart Transplantation in China 172
  6.1 Distribution of medical institutions qualified for heart transplantation 173
  6.2 Demographic characteristics of heart transplant recipients 175
  6.3 Quality and safety analysis of heart transplantation 177
  6.4 Feature and future outlook 179

Chapter 7 Lung Transplantation in China 183
  7.1 Distribution of medical institutions qualified for lung transplantation 184
  7.2 Demographic characteristics of lung transplant recipients 187
  7.3 Quality and safety analysis of lung transplantation 190
  7.4 Feature and future outlook 195

Chapter 8 The Development of Technologies and Innovations for Organ Transplantation in China 199
  8.1 Establishment and promotion of key technical system for split liver transplantation 199
  8.2 The AGH score is a predictor of disease-free survival and targeted therapy efficacy after liver transplantation in patients with hepatocellular carcinoma 202
  8.3 A novel stratification integrating dual biomarkers in liver transplantation for hepatocellular carcinoma 206
  8.4 Establishment and application of core technology system for the treatment of multiple organ failure with natural polymer biological liver materials 208
  8.5 Genotype-guided model used for precise anti-rejection therapy after

	liver transplantation	211
8.6	Application of Da Vinci robot-assisted laparoscopy in kidney transplantation	213
8.7	The utilization of an artificial protective external vascular sheath in renal transplantation represents a novel technological advancement aimed at preventing graft artery kinking	217
8.8	Six-genes edited porcine-rhesus kidney xenotran-splantation	219
8.9	The first group of 37 cases of kidney transplantation for infants and young children in China	221
8.10	Ischemia-free heart transplantation	224
8.11	A novel myocardial biopsy technique after heart transplantation	225
8.12	A machine learning based prognostic model for lung transplant patients	228
8.13	Robot-assisted lung transplantation	230
8.14	Application of donor-derived cell-free DNA in diagnosing rejection after lung transplantation	232

第一章　中国人体器官捐献

器官捐献是挽救垂危生命、弘扬人间大爱的高尚事业。2023年10月20日中华人民共和国国务院第17次常务会议通过的《人体器官捐献和移植条例》，进一步凸显器官捐献的重要性，规定器官捐献要坚持自愿、无偿的原则，依据《中华人民共和国民法典》完善了器官捐献的条件和程序；规定国家加强器官捐献的宣传教育和知识普及，新闻媒体应当开展器官捐献的公益宣传，以此促进形成有利于器官捐献的社会风尚；规定国家鼓励遗体器官捐献，强化褒扬和引导。党中央、国务院高度重视人体器官捐献和移植事业。各级卫生健康部门与红十字会团结协作、积极探索、创新发展，构建并不断完善人体器官捐献工作体系，广泛开展人体器官捐献宣传动员、意愿登记、捐献见证、缅怀纪念、人道关怀等工作，加强人体器官捐献组织网络、协调员队伍建设和管理，取得显著成效。

一、机构和队伍建设情况

1. 工作机构

2023年，吉林、河南、甘肃3个省级红十字会新成立了人体器官捐献管理机构。截至2023年底，全国已有30个省级红十字会成立了人体器官捐献管理机构（表1–1）。

表1-1 2023年底全国省级红十字会人体器官捐献管理机构成立情况

序号	省（自治区、直辖市）	机构名称
1	北京	北京市红十字会捐献服务中心
2	天津	天津市红十字事务中心
3	河北	河北省红十字会三献工作事务中心
4	山西	山西省红十字会社会工作服务中心
5	内蒙古	内蒙古自治区红十字会捐献服务中心
6	辽宁	辽宁省红十字事业发展服务中心
7	吉林	吉林省红十字会捐献服务中心
8	黑龙江	黑龙江省红十字备灾捐献中心
9	上海	上海市红十字事务中心
10	江苏	江苏省人体器官捐献管理中心
11	浙江	浙江省人体器官捐献管理中心
12	安徽	安徽省红十字会捐献办公室
13	福建	福建省人体器官捐献管理中心
14	江西	江西省红十字会人道救助服务中心
15	山东	山东省红十字会医学捐献服务中心
16	河南	河南省人体器官捐献管理办公室
17	湖北	湖北省人体器官捐献管理中心
18	湖南	湖南省人体器官捐献管理中心
19	广东	广东省红十字会器官捐献管理办公室
20	广西	广西壮族自治区人体器官捐献管理中心
21	海南	海南省红十字医学捐献服务中心
22	重庆	重庆市遗体器官捐献管理中心
23	四川	四川省人体器官捐献管理中心
24	贵州	贵州省人体器官与细胞组织捐献管理中心
25	云南	云南省人体器官捐献管理中心
26	陕西	陕西省人体器官捐献管理中心
27	甘肃	甘肃省红十字人道事务服务中心
28	青海	青海省人体器官捐献管理中心
29	宁夏	宁夏回族自治区人体器官捐献服务中心
30	新疆	新疆维吾尔自治区人体器官捐献管理中心

2. 协调员队伍

2023年，中国人体器官捐献管理中心分别在黑龙江省哈尔滨市、山东省临沂市、湖北省武汉市举办了三期全国人体器官捐献协调员培训班，培训新入职协调员400余人。截至2023年底，全国在册协调员2 602人，其中红十字会工作人员1 127人，医疗机构红十字志愿者1 475人（图1-1）。

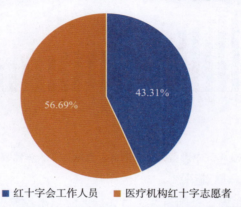

图1-1　截至2023年底全国人体器官捐献协调员构成

3. 能力建设

2023年，中国人体器官捐献管理中心在湖南省长沙市举办了首期人体器官捐献专家学术讲座，各省（自治区、直辖市）红十字会相关负责人、医疗机构代表和有关专家300余人参加；在海南省海口市举办了第七期全国人体器官捐献高级培训班，培训管理人员及业务骨干120余人；在山西省太原市、云南省昆明市举办了两期协调员综合能力建设师资研修班，培训协调员师资70余人。

二、志愿登记情况

1. 志愿登记区域分布

2023年，全国人体器官捐献志愿登记人数新增82万，全国人体器官捐献志愿登记人数达665万。志愿登记人数排名前十位的省（自治区、直辖市）分别为广东（56.8万）、山东（54.29万）、江苏（49.52万）、河南（45.18万）、四川（44.81万）、浙江（34.21万）、安徽（32.28万）、湖北（27.41万）、河北（27.13万）、湖南（25.49万）（图1-2）。

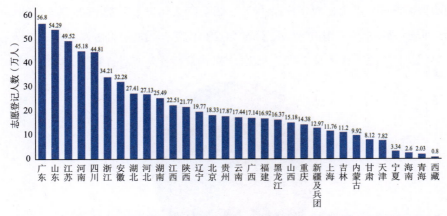

图1-2 截至2023年底中国各省（自治区、直辖市）人体器官捐献志愿登记人数

2. 每万人口志愿登记率

截至2023年底，全国每万人口人体器官捐献志愿登记率为47.2，排名前十位的省（自治区、直辖市）分别为北京（83.9）、江苏（58.1）、天津（57.3）、陕西（55.1）、山东（53.6）、四川（53.5）、安徽（52.7）、上海（52.2）、浙江（51.6）、吉林（50.3）（图1-3）。

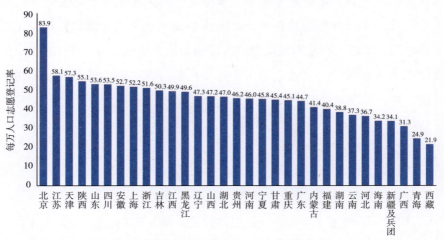

图1-3 截至2023年底中国各省（自治区、直辖市）每万人口人体器官捐献志愿登记率

第一章 中国人体器官捐献

3. 志愿登记者年龄构成

截至2023年底，全国人体器官捐献志愿登记者年龄构成为18～25岁占40%、26～35岁占38.2%、36～45岁占14.6%、46～60岁占5.6%、>60岁占1.6%（图1-4），中青年登记者占大多数。

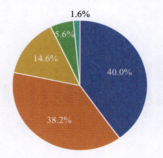

图1-4 截至2023年底全国人体器官捐献志愿登记者年龄构成

三、器官捐献情况

1. 年捐献量

2023年，中国遗体器官捐献例数6 454例，较2022年增长14.39%；自2010年以来，遗体器官捐献例数累计达4.9万余例，累计捐献大器官15.3万余个。2023年遗体器官捐献例数前十位的省（自治区、直辖市）分别为广东（774例）、山东（669例）、广西（561例）、湖北（462例）、北京（419例）、湖南（314例）、河南（310例）、浙江（283例）、陕西（280例）、四川（245例）（图1-5）。

2. 每百万人口捐献率

2023年，全国每百万人口遗体器官捐献率（organ donation per million population，PMP）为4.58，PMP排名前十位的省（自治区、直辖市）分别为北京（19.2）、海南（11.4）、广西（11.2）、湖北（7.9）、吉林（7.4）、陕西（7.1）、山东（6.6）、广东（6.1）、辽宁（5.4）、重庆（5.2）（图1-6）。

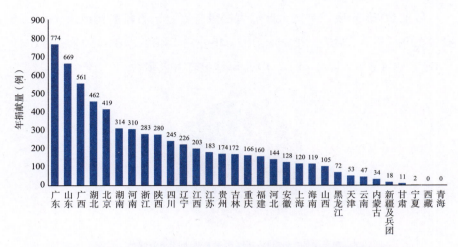

图 1-5　2023 年中国各省（自治区、直辖市）遗体器官捐献例数

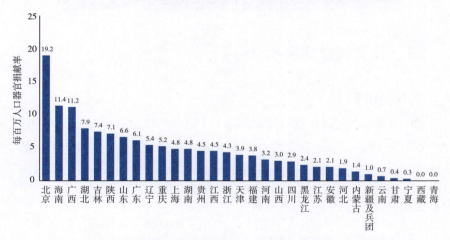

图 1-6　2023 年中国各省（自治区、直辖市）遗体器官捐献 PMP

3. 器官捐献者性别构成

2023 年，中国遗体器官捐献者以男性为主，占比为 81.05%，女性占 18.95%（图 1-7）。

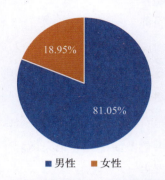

图 1-7 2023 年中国遗体器官捐献者性别构成

四、相关工作开展

2023 年，在国家卫生健康委员会、中国红十字会总会指导和支持下，中国人体器官捐献管理中心、中国器官移植发展基金会等机构积极推进器官捐献理念宣传、器官捐献志愿登记、器官捐献工作见证、志愿服务体系建设及活动开展等相关工作，不断建立完善人体器官捐献相关工作机制。

1. 宣传动员与公益活动

2023 年，开展多场面对公众的主题宣传活动。制作《生命·遇见》宣传册和《一个人的力量》《生命接力·大爱传递》宣传片，推动《一个人的球队》《生死摆渡》电影创作。在江西南昌举办首届人体器官捐献"生命接力"运动会，在全国发起人体器官捐献生命接力"云"动会，以"互联网＋运动打卡＋理念传播"形式开展活动，设 31 个赛区，累计 436 个团队、4.9 万余人参加。在全国发起"生命之约·大爱传递"——全国人体器官捐献志愿登记宣传季活动，推动各地红十字会开展 100 余场器官捐献宣传进医院、进高校、进企业、进社区等活动。开展 31 次生命接力先锋队联学联建主题党日活动，"生命接力万里行"健步走宣传活动；第七个中国器官捐献主题宣传活动全国近 200 家单位参与，活动总传播量 3 亿，当日相关微博话题排热搜第 9 位。开展"生命接力 百城行动"公益项目系列活动，在 12 个城市持续、广泛、多形式宣传器官捐献理念。

2. 志愿登记与咨询服务

2023年人体器官捐献志愿登记人数新增82万人，接听咨询电话2.4万余次，回复咨询短信8 500余人次，处理咨询邮件1 100余件，制作发放志愿登记实体卡和感谢信60余万套。继续拓展器官捐献志愿登记渠道，其中施予受器官捐献志愿者服务系统已与133家合作单位完成技术对接，为有捐献意愿的民众提供更多便捷的登记渠道。

3. 捐献见证与案例报告

2023年完成人体器官捐献见证6 454例，坚持"自愿、无偿"原则，现场见证并客观记录捐献确认、器官获取和分配过程及结果，通过中国人体器官捐献案例报告管理系统及时准确填报捐献案例相关信息，维护捐献者及其家属的相关权益。

4. 缅怀纪念与人道关怀

在全国发起主题为"生命·遇见"人体器官捐献缅怀纪念月活动，在湖南长沙举办2023全国人体器官捐献缅怀纪念暨宣传普及活动，同步组织举办云上缅怀纪念活动，致敬捐献者及其家属的大爱奉献精神。在山西阳泉、浙江乐清、广东汕头等地新建缅怀纪念场所29个，向每户人体器官捐献者家庭颁发捐献证书、纪念章和慰问信，广泛开展回访慰问、心理抚慰、子女助学等关怀活动。发挥中国器官移植发展基金会等慈善组织的使命和责任，凝聚社会爱心，对困难的器官捐献者家庭实施慈善救助，形成全社会团结互助的社会风尚，培育符合中国国情的捐献文化与社会氛围。

5. 志愿服务体系建设

召开人体器官捐献志愿服务暨文艺创作研讨会，筹备成立中国人体器官捐献志愿服务工作委员会。在全国发起人体器官捐献志愿服务月活动，支持开展"小桔灯""天使爱妈妈"等10个人体器官捐献志愿服务项目。截至2023年底，在全国建立人体器官捐献志愿服务队600余支，志愿者人数达2万余人。成立全国卫生健康行业器官捐献青年志愿服务总队，面向全国卫生健康行业、高等院校等器官捐献相关领域招募青年志愿者，以实际行动助力器官捐献事业健康发展。

6. 传播与信息平台建设

编印《中国人体器官捐献工作通讯》12期，向全国700余家单位和个人发放。截至2023年底，"中国人体器官捐献"微信公众号关注人数达530余万人。新开通"中国人体器官捐献"支付宝生活号和喜马拉雅主播号。改版升级中国人体器官捐献管理中心网站、微网站，升级人体器官捐献志愿登记和案例报告管理系统。中国器官移植发展基金会自媒体传播矩阵关注总人数165.5万余人；每月形成月报发送至132家器官捐献志愿服务合作单位，就工作开展情况进行统计信息同步。完成与中国人体器官分配与共享计算机系统（China Organ Transplant Response System，COTRS）的对接，实现潜在器官捐献者志愿登记信息自动核验功能。

五、工作展望

全面贯彻落实《人体器官捐献和移植条例》，计划制定出台捐献见证、人道关怀等相关配套文件，继续推动人体器官捐献法规制度和工作机制建设，不断提升人体器官捐献工作法治化、专业化、规范化水平。加强协调员队伍建设、管理和服务，为协调员开展工作提供更有力的保障。大力开展宣传动员，支持各地举办特色宣传活动，推进人体器官捐献宣传进医院、进高校、进社区、进企业，继续推动拓宽器官捐献志愿登记渠道。继续组织举办全国人体器官捐献缅怀纪念暨宣传普及活动，继续推动具备条件的县级以上城市建设捐献者缅怀纪念设施，推动省级红十字会建立完善人道关怀工作机制，进一步营造鼓励器官捐献大爱奉献精神的社会氛围。

第二章　中国人体捐献器官获取

数据范围介绍

中国人体捐献器官获取章节内容数据来源于 COTRS 和人体器官获取组织（Organ Procurement Organization，OPO）基础信息库，涵盖 OPO 组织架构、队伍建设以及人体捐献器官获取数据，统计周期为 2023 年 1 月 1 日至 12 月 31 日。

统计方法介绍

本章节数据均采用描述性统计分析方法。

章节要点

（1）截至 2023 年底，中国共有 109 个 OPO，全国 OPO 工作人员为 1 261 人，平均每个 OPO 配置工作人员 12 人。

（2）2023 年全国有 20 个 OPO 年捐献量≥100 例，其总量占中国年捐献量的 53.24%。

（3）脑死亡来源器官捐献者占比逐年提升；每供体获取器官数有所提升，获取器官利用率较 2022 年略有下降；捐献器官移植原发性无功能（primary nonfunction，PNF）发生率和移植后功能延迟性恢复（delayed graft function，DGF）发生率保持在较高水平。

（4）下一步，将继续加强医疗机构 OPO 学科体系建设，全面推进人体器官捐献源头培训，推动人体捐献器官获取能力持续提升，启动器官捐献及获取能力评估工作，共筑医疗行业器官捐献发展新格局。

一、人体捐献器官获取体系建设与发展

2014年3月1日,在国务院的领导下,中国人体器官捐献与移植委员会成立。中国人体器官捐献与移植"五大工作体系":人体器官捐献体系、人体器官获取与分配体系、人体器官移植临床服务体系、人体器官获取与移植质控体系和人体器官捐献与移植监管体系正式构建,由中国人体器官捐献与移植委员会统筹指导。

人体捐献器官获取是五大工作体系中从人体器官捐献到人体器官分配的重要工作环节,是从器官捐献到器官移植前各项必不可少的流程总和;由OPO承担主要工作,其工作人员包括器官捐献协调员、专职医师、专职护士、数据报送员及管理人员等,工作内容涵盖宣传动员、潜在器官捐献者识别转介、捐献者抢救维护与评估、申请死亡判定、协助完成器官捐献伦理、捐献器官获取、捐献者善后处理等。

2015年,中国实现公民自愿器官捐献的全面转型,自此,中国器官捐献与移植事业进入高速发展的新时期。2016年起,中国遗体器官捐献量稳定保持在世界第二位,亚洲第一位。2015—2023年,中国累计完成遗体器官捐献4.67万例,捐献大器官突破14.02万个。

2023年12月14日,《人体器官捐献和移植条例》(以下简称《条例》)发布,进一步凸显器官捐献的重要性,强化对器官捐献的褒扬和引导,将全面促进我国器官捐献与移植事业高质量可持续发展。《条例》对器官获取与分配管理作出详细规定,明确了省级政府卫生健康部门的监管职责、医疗机构从事遗体器官获取的具体条件以及医疗机构报告器官捐献信息的有关要求。《条例》明确了器官获取医疗机构基本要求、器官获取成本及收费管理要求、质控要求等,并提出了对捐献人和获取的器官进行医学检查、开展移植风险评估等要求。

2023年,按照国家卫生健康委员会有关要求,国家人体捐献器官获取质量控制中心(National Quality Control Center for Donated Organ

Procurement，OPQC）通过三级质控网络建设，积极完善人体捐献器官获取质控体系；开展"器官获取质量行"专项调研，持续推动 OPO 规范管理与能力提升；启动人体器官捐献源头师资培训，全面助推二级及以上医疗机构器官捐献工作。

二、OPO 机构分布与建设情况

1. 机构分布

截至 2023 年底，中国有 109 个 OPO，其中全省统一 OPO（独立法人）1 个、全省统一 OPO（挂靠医疗机构）6 个、联合 OPO 22 个、医疗机构 OPO 80 个（图 2-1）。按照全省统一 OPO 管理的省（自治区、直辖市）有山西、吉林、天津、海南、浙江、江苏、云南，实行联合 OPO 管理的省（自治区、直辖市）有广东、北京、湖南、上海、河北、福建、黑龙江。

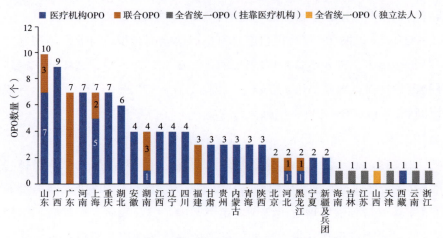

图 2-1　2023 年中国各省（自治区、直辖市）OPO 数量及运行模式

2. 队伍建设

配备充足的工作人员是保障人体捐献器官获取工作的前提。结合 OPO 基础信息库来看，2023 年人体捐献器官获取工作人员 1 261 人，平均每个 OPO 配置工作人员 12 人。29.63% 的 OPO 配置工作人员 < 6 人，

44.44% 的 OPO 配置工作人员在 6~12 人之间，25.93% 的 OPO 配置工作人员 > 12 人。

三、器官捐献情况

1. 总体情况

2023 年有 20 个 OPO 年捐献量 ≥ 100 例，其总量占中国年捐献量的 53.24%（表 2-1）。

表 2-1　2023 年中国年捐献量排名前 20 的 OPO

地区	OPO 名称	年捐献量(例)	运行模式 *
浙江	浙江省人体器官获取服务管理中心	283	2
北京	北部联合体人体器官获取组织	275	3
广西	广西医科大学第二附属医院人体器官获取组织	267	4
陕西	西安交通大学第一附属医院 OPO	238	4
广东	广东省第一 OPO	194	3
四川	四川大学华西医院人体器官获取组织	194	4
江苏	江苏省人体器官获取服务管理中心	183	2
广东	广东省第二 OPO	182	3
吉林	吉林大学第一医院人体器官获取组织	172	2
湖南	湖南省人体器官获取组织第二组	162	3
河南	郑州大学第一附属医院 OPO	158	4
北京	南部联合体人体器官获取组织	144	3
山东	青岛大学附属医院联合 OPO	141	3
湖北	武汉大学中南医院人体器官获取组织	140	4
河北	河北省人体器官获取组织第二工作组	136	3
湖北	华中科技大学同济医学院附属同济医院人体器官获取组织	134	4
海南	海南省人体器官获取组织	119	2
山东	山东省千佛山医院 OPO	107	4
山西	山西省人体器官获取与分配服务中心	105	1
辽宁	解放军北部战区总医院 OPO	102	4

注：组织形式 1. 全省统一 OPO（独立法人）；2. 全省统一 OPO（挂靠医疗机构）；3. 联合 OPO；4. 医疗机构 OPO。

2. 器官捐献分类占比

2023年中国脑死亡供体（donors after brain death，DBD）占比70.70%；心脏死亡供体（donors after circulatory death，DCD）占比21.71%；脑–心双死亡供体（donors after brain and circulatory death，DBCD）占比7.59%（图2-2）。与2022年相比，DBD占比上升3.96个百分点。

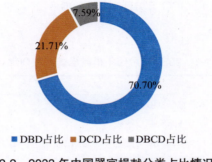

图2-2　2023年中国器官捐献分类占比情况

四、器官获取与利用情况

2023年，全国OPO获取遗体捐献器官20 854个，较2022年增长15.71%，每供体获取器官数为3.23，较2022年有一定提升。每供体获取肝脏、肾脏、心脏、肺脏数分别为0.92、1.87、0.16、0.28；每供体获取肝脏和肾脏数与2022年（0.93，1.88）相比略有下降，每供体获取心脏和肺脏数与2022年（0.13，0.26）相比有所上升（图2-3）。9个省（自治区、直辖市）每供体获取器官数超过全国水平（图2-4）。

2023年，中国获取器官利用率为96.55%，低于2022年（96.74%）。获取肝脏利用率95.99%，获取肾脏利用率96.84%，获取心脏利用率96.10%，获取肺脏利用率96.71%（图2-5）。14个省（自治区、直辖市）获取器官利用率超过全国水平，内蒙古、甘肃和宁夏获取器官利用率为100%（图2-6）。

第二章 中国人体捐献器官获取

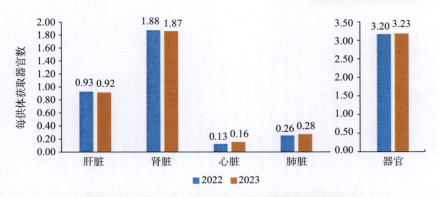

图 2-3 2022 年和 2023 年中国每供体获取器官数

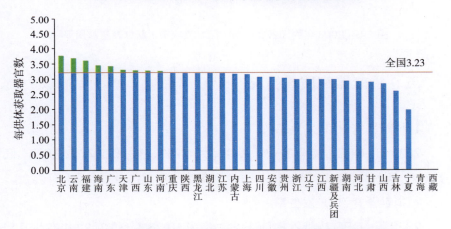

图 2-4 2023 年中国各省（自治区、直辖市）每供体获取器官数

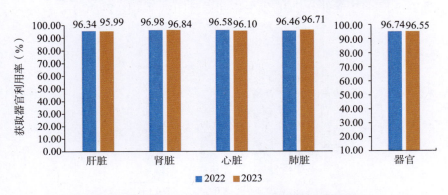

图 2-5 2022 年和 2023 年中国获取器官利用率

15

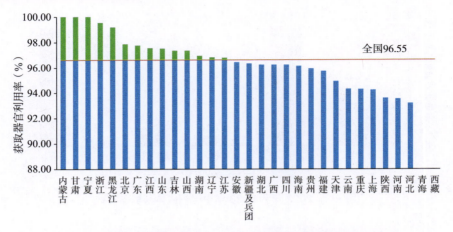

图 2-6　2023 年中国各省（自治区、直辖市）获取器官利用率

五、捐献器官质量情况

1. 捐献器官 PNF 发生率

2023 年，OPO 捐献器官 PNF 发生率为 1.20%，较 2022 年有所升高，低于 2021 年水平（图 2-7）。10 个省份 PNF 发生率超过全国水平（图 2-8）。

2. 捐献器官 DGF 发生率

2023 年，OPO 捐献器官 DGF 发生率为 10.25%，较 2022 年有所升高（图 2-9）。10 个省份 DGF 发生率超过全国水平（图 2-10）。

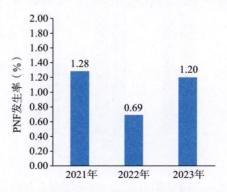

图 2-7　近 3 年中国 PNF 发生率变化情况

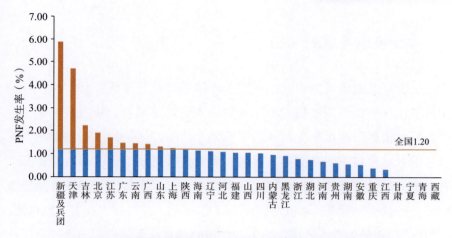

图 2-8　2023 年中国各省（自治区、直辖市）PNF 发生率

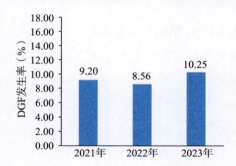

图 2-9　近 3 年中国 DGF 发生率变化情况

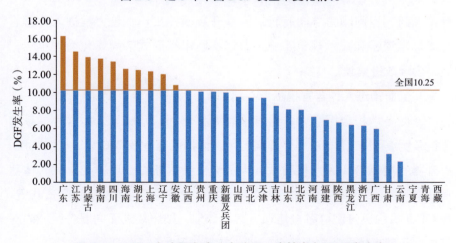

图 2-10　2023 年中国各省（自治区、直辖市）DGF 发生率

六、特点与展望

在国家卫生健康委员会、中国人体器官捐献与移植委员会的领导和支持下，器官捐献与移植"中国模式"实现高速发展。特别是近年来，随着器官捐献与移植相关政策的不断健全、质控体系的不断完善，中国器官捐献与移植事业从高速发展向高质量发展稳步迈进。从数据情况来看，年捐献量持续增长，已超过历史最高水平。捐献器官获取数量稳步提升，捐献器官质量及移植预后保持较高水平，OPO技术能力不断增强。作为拥有14亿人口的大国，中国人体捐献器官获取管理与质量控制将从以下4个方面继续展开。

1. 加强医疗机构OPO学科体系建设

按照《人体器官捐献和移植条例》有关要求，坚持人体捐献器官获取事业高质量发展的原则，秉持创新模式、精准质控的科学管理理念，有序推进器官获取专业学科建设，着力完善OPO组织架构，加强人体捐献器官获取场地设施建设、设备投入及人员培养，建立长效管理机制，严格落实医疗核心制度，建立捐献器官获取临床诊疗常规，科学开展器官功能维护、器官质量评估与质量控制。持续开展"器官获取质量行"专项调研，以问题为导向有针对性地开展质控工作，着力推进人体器官获取标准流程和技术规范实施，研讨不同组织形式下同质化管理难点，提出合理改进建议。

2. 全面推进人体器官捐献源头培训

督促各地积极组织人体器官捐献源头培训，开展《人体器官捐献和移植条例》宣贯工作，进一步提高各地人体捐献器官获取政策法规知晓度，提升器官捐献源头医疗机构医务人员专业技术能力，培养专业化人体器官获取团队。OPQC负责进行人体器官捐献源头师资培训，组建师资队伍；各OPO机构负责制订各自培训方案与计划，按照要求面向服务区域内医疗机构开展人体器官捐献源头培训，持续提升地区PMP。

3. 推动人体捐献器官获取能力持续提升

加强 OPO 机构器官获取能力建设，落实捐献器官获取伦理审查，推进捐献者微生物感染基因测序及器官保存液病原微生物培养、微生物基因测序，开展捐献器官病理活检，同时加强器官质量优化的临床转化研究，促进体外膜氧合（extracorporeal membrane oxygenation，ECMO）、机械灌注等特色技术发展，有力保障捐献器官质量。

4. 启动器官捐献及获取能力评估工作

开展 OPO 器官获取及能力评估工作，不断强化 OPO 建设与管理。同时将能力评估工作延伸至服务区域二级及以上医疗机构，建立二级及以上器官捐献工作台账，溯源器官捐献来源医院情况，不断提升捐献器官获取质量，全面推进二级及以上医疗机构器官捐献工作开展，共筑医疗行业器官捐献发展新格局。

第三章　中国人体器官分配与共享

数据范围介绍

中国人体器官分配与共享章节内容数据来源于COTRS，选取2015年1月1日至2023年12月31日的数据。

统计方法介绍

对器官捐献和移植等待者的基本情况采用描述性统计分析。

章节要点

（1）2023年中国完成人体器官捐献10 778例，其中遗体器官捐献6 454例（59.88%）、亲属间活体捐献4 324例（40.12%），实施器官移植手术23 905例，其中遗体器官捐献来源19 581例（81.91%）、亲属间活体器官捐献4 324例（18.09%），包括多器官联合移植119例，同期有160 767人等待器官移植。

（2）2023年中国遗体器官捐献者年龄中位数为49岁，儿童捐献者（＜18岁）共478例，占7.41%；从捐献分类来看，70.70%为脑死亡器官捐献；脑血管意外为主要死亡原因，占53.59%。

（3）2023年共有160 767人在等待名单中，包括肾脏134 011人、肝脏21 940人、心脏3 182人、肺脏1 634人。2023年末，有45 212人不再等待器官移植，仍有115 555名器官衰竭患者等待移植，其中等待肾脏、肝脏、心脏和肺脏移植的人数分别为105 458人、8 288人、1 457人和352人。

第三章　中国人体器官分配与共享

自2015年1月1日至2023年12月31日,中国遗体器官捐献(deceased donation, DD)累计完成46 688例,PMP从2015年的2.01上升至2023年的4.58。2023年,中国完成人体器官捐献10 778例,其中遗体器官捐献6 454例(59.88%)、亲属间活体捐献4 324例(40.12%),实施器官移植手术23 905例,其中遗体器官捐献来源19 581例(81.91%)、亲属间活体器官捐献4 324例(18.09%),包括多器官联合移植119例。

《人体器官移植条例》自2007年施行以来,对促进人体器官公平分配发挥了重要的作用,我国已初步建成符合世界卫生组织《人体细胞、组织和器官移植指导原则》等国际通行原则的人体器官获取与分配制度体系。2013年启用COTRS自动分配遗体捐献器官,有效保障了器官分配的科学、公平、公正、公开。2018年国家卫生健康委员会对《卫生部关于印发中国人体器官分配与共享基本原则和肝脏与肾脏移植核心政策的通知》(卫医管发〔2010〕113号)进行了修订,并制定了心脏、肺脏分配与共享核心政策,形成了《中国人体器官分配与共享基本原则和核心政策》(以下简称"器官分配核心政策")。

2023年,新修订的《人体器官捐献和移植条例》将人体器官获取与分配管理有关规定由部门的规范性文件上升为行政法规,为人体器官获取与分配管理提供了法治保障,器官获取与分配体系建设必将更加法治化、专业化、科学化,器官捐献与移植事业也必将更加公平、可持续和高质量发展,人民群众健康权益将得到进一步维护。

COTRS是中国器官捐献与移植工作体系的重要组成部分,由"潜在器官捐献者识别系统""人体器官捐献人登记及器官匹配系统""人体器官移植等待者预约名单系统"3个子系统及监管平台组成。作为执行中国器官分配与共享相关法律法规和科学政策的专用系统,COTRS执行国家器官科学分配政策,实施自动器官分配和共享,并向国家和地方监管机构提供全程监控,建立器官获取和分配的溯源性,最大限度地排除人为干预,保障器官分配的公平、公正、公开,是中国遗体器官捐献工作赢得人民群众信任的重要基石。

一、中国移植医疗机构分布

截至2023年12月31日，中国有188所具有器官移植资质的医疗机构，较2022年新增5所，各省（自治区、直辖市）移植医疗机构分布见图3-1。其中，数量排名居前十位的省（自治区、直辖市）为广东（21所）、北京（17所）、上海（13所）、山东（12所）、福建（10所）、湖南（10所）、浙江（10所）、湖北（8所）、河南（7所）和江苏（7所）。

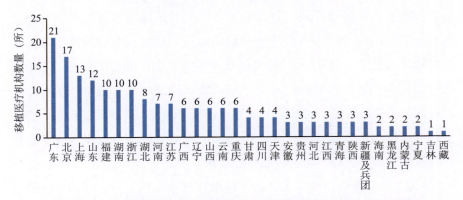

图3-1　2023年中国各省（自治区、直辖市）移植医疗机构分布情况

二、人体器官捐献情况

1. 人体器官捐献量

2015—2023年，中国遗体器官捐献量和PMP稳步提升，从2015年2 766例上升至2023年6 454例，PMP从2015年2.01上升至2023年4.58（图3-2）。2020—2023年，中国遗体器官捐献量保持平稳增长（图3-3）。

2. 器官捐献者特征

2023年，中国遗体器官捐献者年龄中位数为49岁，儿童捐献者（＜18岁）共478例，占7.41%，其中＜2岁捐献者87例（18.20%），2～6岁捐献者103例（21.55%），7～13岁捐献者132例（27.62%），

14~18岁捐献者156例（32.64%）。捐献者以男性为主，占比为81.05%。捐献者的血型以O型为主，占37.08%；其次是A型和B型，分别占28.60%和25.98%；AB型占8.34%（图3-4）。70.70%为中国Ⅰ类（脑死亡器官捐献），21.71%为中国Ⅱ类（心脏死亡器官捐献），7.59%为中国Ⅲ类（脑-心死亡器官捐献）（图3-5）。

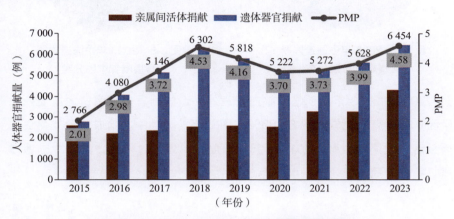

图3-2　2015—2023年中国人体器官捐献量

注：2015—2019年人口数来自《中国卫生健康统计年鉴》，2020—2023年人口数来源于国家统计局。

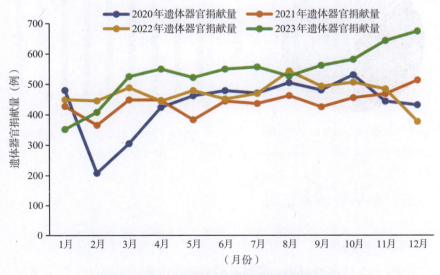

图3-3　2023年中国遗体器官捐献量变化趋势

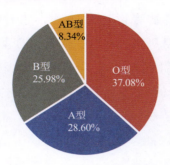 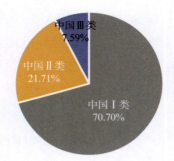

图 3-4　2023 年中国遗体器官捐献者血型分布

图 3-5　2023 年中国遗体器官捐献者中国分类

2015—2023 年，创伤和脑血管意外为遗体器官捐献者两大主要死亡原因，占所有死亡原因的 86.85%（图 3-6）。其中，脑血管意外死亡的捐献者占比逐年上升。2019 年起，脑血管意外超过创伤，成为中国遗体器官捐献者的首要死亡原因（图 3-7）。

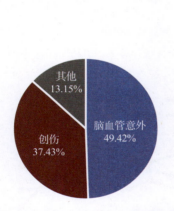 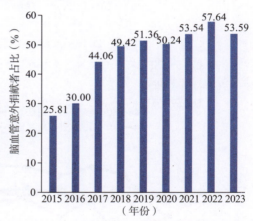

图 3-6　2015—2023 年中国遗体器官捐献者死亡原因占比

图 3-7　2015—2023 年中国遗体器官捐献者脑血管意外占比

三、移植等待者情况

1. 移植等待量

2015—2023 年，肝脏、肾脏移植等待者数量（图 3-8）逐年增加。

第三章 中国人体器官分配与共享

2023年共有160 767名器官衰竭患者等待器官移植,包括肾脏移植等待者134 011人、肝脏移植等待者21 940人、心脏移植等待者3 182人、肺脏移植等待者1 634人。目前,中国尚未建立全国统一的胰腺、小肠移植等待名单。同期,中国有23 905人(14.87%)接受器官移植手术(图3-9)。

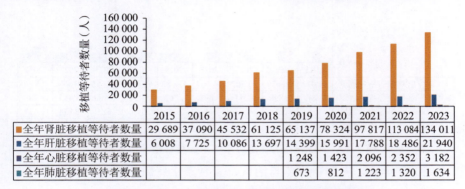

	2015	2016	2017	2018	2019	2020	2021	2022	2023
全年肾脏移植等待者数量	29 689	37 090	45 532	61 125	65 137	78 324	97 817	113 084	134 011
全年肝脏移植等待者数量	6 008	7 725	10 086	13 697	14 399	15 991	17 788	18 486	21 940
全年心脏移植等待者数量					1 248	1 423	2 096	2 352	3 182
全年肺脏移植等待者数量					673	812	1 223	1 320	1 634

图 3-8　2015—2023年历年器官移植等待者数量

	移植总量	肝脏移植	肾脏移植	心脏移植	肺脏移植	胰腺移植	小肠移植
2015	10 057	2 620	7 040	279	118		
2016	13 263	3 672	9 019	368	204		
2017	16 687	5 149	10 793	446	299		
2018	20 201	6 279	13 029	490	403		
2019	19 454	6 170	12 124	679	489		
2020	17 897	5 842	11 037	557	513		
2021	19 326	5 834	12 039	738	775		
2022	20 333	6 053	12 712	710	798	45	15
2023	23 905	6 896	14 968	994	959	76	12

图 3-9　2015—2023年历年器官移植数量

注 其中2019—2023年分别涉及8例、52例、60例、89例及119例多器官联合移植。

2. 年末移植等待情况

2023年末,中国仍有115 555名器官衰竭患者等待移植,其中105 458人等待肾脏移植、8 288人等待肝脏移植、1 457人等待心脏移植,352人等待肺脏移植(图3-10)。有45 212人不再等待器官移植,原因包括已实施器官移植手术、身体状态明显改善不需进行器官移植手术、病情严重不能接受移植手术、死亡等。

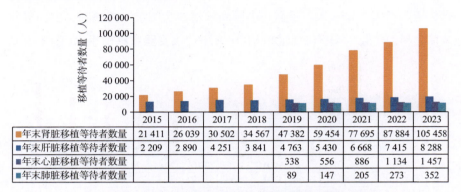

图3-10 2015—2023年历年年末器官移植等待者数量

2023年末，中国各省（自治区、直辖市）肾脏移植等待者数量分布见图3-11，其中排名前十位的省（自治区、直辖市）分别为浙江（13 322人）、广东（13 314人）、湖南（8 837人）、河南（8 136人）、四川（7 665人）、上海（6 921人）、湖北（6 038人）、广西（5 439人）、山东（3 589人）和北京（3 401人）。

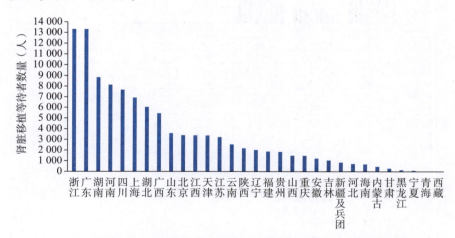

图3-11 2023年末中国各省（自治区、直辖市）肾脏移植等待者数量

2023年末，中国各省（自治区、直辖市）肝脏移植等待者数量分布见图3-12，其中排名前十位的省（自治区、直辖市）分别为四川（1 775

人)、广东(1032人)、浙江(748人)、北京(594人)、天津(488人)、上海(477人)、江苏(421人)、湖北(397人)、湖南(341人)和云南(320人)。

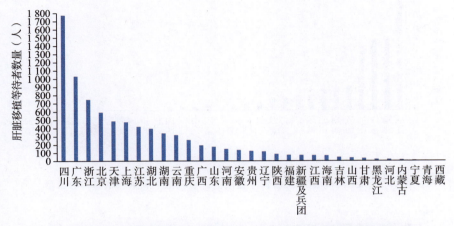

图 3-12　2023 年末中国各省(自治区、直辖市)肝脏移植等待者数量

2023 年末,中国各省(自治区、直辖市)心脏移植等待者数量分布见图 3-13,其中排名前十位的省(自治区、直辖市)分别为北京(339人)、湖北(281人)、河南(142人)、广东(107人)、上海(97人)、浙江(91人)、湖南(72人)、陕西(52人)、山东(41人)和四川(38人)。

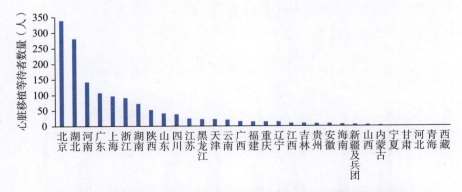

图 3-13　2023 年末中国各省(自治区、直辖市)心脏移植等待者数量

2023 年末,中国各省(自治区、直辖市)肺脏移植等待者数量分布见图 3-14,其中排名前十位的省(自治区、直辖市)分别为浙江(82人)、湖北（53人）、广东（52人）、河南（44人）、安徽（18人）、湖南（18人）、四川（18人）、陕西（11人）、上海（11人）、北京（9人）和江苏（9人）。

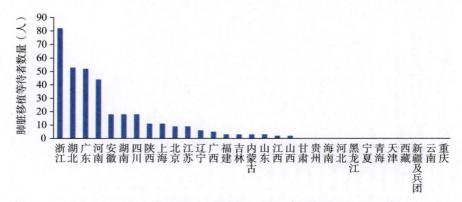

图3-14　2023年末中国各省（自治区、直辖市）肺脏移植等待者数量

四、人体器官分配与共享政策实施效果

1. 遗体器官捐献者获取器官数进一步提高

2015—2023年，每位遗体器官捐献者平均获取器官数平稳增长，如肝脏平均获取器官数从2015年0.88个上升至2023年0.92个。心脏、肺脏平均获取器官数持续提升，2023年，心脏平均获取器官数为0.16个，肺脏平均获取器官数为0.28个（图3-15）。

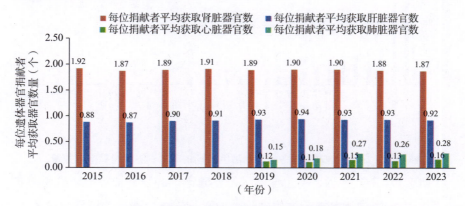

图3-15　2015—2023年每位遗体器官捐献者平均获取的器官数

第三章 中国人体器官分配与共享

2. 儿童肾脏移植受益显著提高

2018年，国家卫生健康委员会修订的器官分配核心政策，进一步全面推进和贯彻优先保障儿童利益、推动公共资源优先向儿童配置的原则，结合肾脏疾病和透析治疗给少年儿童生长发育带来的严重不良影响，小于18岁捐献者的肾脏优先分配给小于18岁肾脏移植等待者，增加了儿童肾脏移植等待者获得移植的可能性。

比较器官分配核心政策修订前后儿童肾脏移植的情况显示，政策实施后，肾脏移植等待者中获得器官分配的儿童比例呈明显上升趋势。2023年儿童、成人肾脏移植等待者中获得器官分配的比例分别为31.22%、8.29%，儿童肾脏移植等待者获得分配的比例为成人的3.8倍，儿童肾脏移植等待者受益明显。

3. 绿色通道政策促进器官共享

2016年5月6日，国家卫生和计划生育委员会等6部门联合印发了《关于建立人体捐献器官转运绿色通道的通知》（以下简称《通知》），建立人体捐献器官转运绿色通道，《通知》明确了各方职责，目的是确保人体捐献器官转运流程的通畅，将器官转运环节对器官移植患者的质量安全影响减少到最低程度。

《通知》将器官转运分为一般流程及应急流程，转运过程中根据实际情况启动不同流程，实现人体捐献器官转运的快速通关与优先承运，提高转运效率，保障转运安全，减少因运输原因造成的器官浪费。

比较人体捐献器官转运绿色通道政策实施前后中国人体器官共享情况，结果显示，政策实施后，2023年中国器官省内共享比例和全国共享比例分别较政策实施前上升8.4个百分点和2.0个百分点（表3-1）。

表3-1 绿色通道政策实施前后中国器官共享率

共享范围	不同时间段器官共享率（%）			
	政策前	2022年	2023年	变化（2023年与政策前）
OPO共享	75.0	64.2	64.6	−10.4
省内共享	12.6	20.6	21.0	8.4▲
全国共享	12.4	15.1	14.4	2.0▲

注：▲表示有所上升。

五、特点与展望

器官移植是人类医学发展的巨大成就，挽救了无数终末期疾病患者的生命。2023年中国器官捐献、移植数量均位居世界第二。COTRS在执行国家器官科学分配政策，保障器官分配的公平、公正、公开等方面，发挥了重要作用。

1. 人体器官捐献工作平稳有序、分配工作高效规范

2023年，全国共开展遗体器官捐献6 454例、平均器官获取率3.25%、获取器官利用率96.33%，人体器官捐献量创历史新高，人体器官捐献工作平稳有序、分配工作高效规范。同时，全国16.08万名器官移植等待者仅开展23 905例器官移植手术，器官短缺依然是制约我国器官移植事业发展的主要原因。下一步，应继续加大人体器官捐献的宣传力度，强化宣传效果，提升人体器官捐献数量。

2. 保障科学公平，推动人体器官分配法治化建设

新《条例》明确规定，"遗体器官应当通过国务院卫生健康部门建立的分配系统统一分配""从事遗体器官获取、移植的医疗机构应当在分配系统中如实录入遗体器官捐献人、申请人体器官移植手术患者的相关医学数据并及时更新，不得伪造、篡改数据"，并要求"医疗机构及其医务人员应当执行分配系统分配结果"，不得"使用未经分配系统分配的遗体器官或者来源不明的人体器官实施人体器官移植"。这一系列规定，对器官分配流程、关键环节及分配结果的应用均提出了明确的规范和要求。

此外，划定了遗体器官分配的红线，为打击违法违规行为、维护捐献者和移植等待者的合法权益提供了法律依据，有助于规范器官分配，促进我国器官捐献与移植工作健康、可持续发展。同时，《条例》规定，"国务院卫生健康部门应当定期公布遗体器官捐献和分配情况"，主动接受社会监督，提高公众对器官捐献与移植领域的了解，鼓励更多的群众参与遗体器官捐献，挽救更多患者。

3. 开展全国人体器官分配与共享政策修订

为深入开展学习贯彻习近平新时代中国特色社会主义思想主题教育，推动调查研究向纵深开展，提升我国器官分配政策的科学性、先进性，促进我国器官捐献与移植事业高质量发展，COTRS 科学委员会将持续开展全国人体器官分配与共享政策调研活动，共同探讨人体器官捐献与移植临床需求和政策建议。

第四章 中国肝脏移植

数据范围介绍

中国肝脏移植章节内容数据来源于中国肝移植注册系统（China Liver Transplant Registry，CLTR），选取2015年1月1日至2023年12月31日的数据。

统计方法介绍

对肝脏移植受体的基本情况采用描述性统计分析，采用Kaplan-Meier法进行生存分析。

章节要点

（1）2023年，中国肝脏移植例数创历史新高，共实施肝脏移植手术6 896例，较2022年增长13.9%；2023年，有12所医疗机构实施的肝脏移植例数≥150例，其移植总量占全国当年总例数的42.9%；截至2023年底，具备肝脏移植资质的医疗机构达到118所。

（2）中国肝脏移植的平均冷缺血时间、平均无肝期、术中平均失血量、术中平均输红细胞量、平均手术时间等质量指标整体呈逐年改善趋势。

（3）中国儿童肝脏移植稳步发展，积极拓展供肝来源，持续推动肝脏移植医疗质量和服务水平提升。

第四章 中国肝脏移植

一、肝脏移植医疗机构分布

截至2023年12月31日，中国共有118所具有肝脏移植资质的医疗机构。其中，肝脏移植医疗机构数量前十位的省（自治区、直辖市）为北京（13所）、广东（12所）、上海（10所）、山东（8所）、福建（7所）、浙江（7所）、湖北（6所）、广西（5所）、湖南（5所）、重庆（5所）（图4-1）。

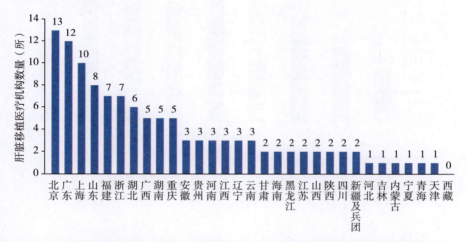

图4-1 2023年中国各省（自治区、直辖市）具有肝脏移植资质的医疗机构地区分布

2015—2023年，中国共实施肝脏移植48 515例，包括41 866例遗体器官捐献肝脏移植（deceased donor liver transplantation，DDLT），占比86.3%；6 649例亲属间活体肝脏移植（living-related donor liver transplantation，LDLT），占比13.7%（图4-2）。成人肝脏移植39 802例，占比82.0%；儿童肝脏移植8 713例，占比18.0%。

2023年，中国共实施肝脏移植手术6 896例，包括5 972例DDLT，占比86.6%；924例LDLT（包括6例多米诺肝脏移植），占比13.4%。成人肝脏移植5 687例，占比82.5%；儿童肝脏移植1 209例，占比17.5%。2023年实施肝脏移植例数排名前十位的省（自治区、直辖市）依次为上海（1 208 例）、浙江（746 例）、广东（666 例）、北京（557 例）、山东（481 例）、湖北（345 例）、广西（336 例）、四川（261 例）、河南（241 例）、天津（241 例）；2023 年实施≥100 例肝脏移植的省（自治区、直辖市）有 20 个，移植总量占中国当年肝脏移植总例数的 94.9%（图 4-3）；青海和西藏在 2023 年未开展肝脏移植。

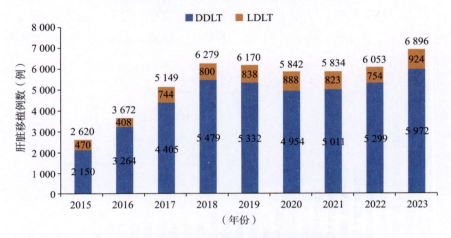

图 4-2　2015—2023 年中国肝脏移植例数

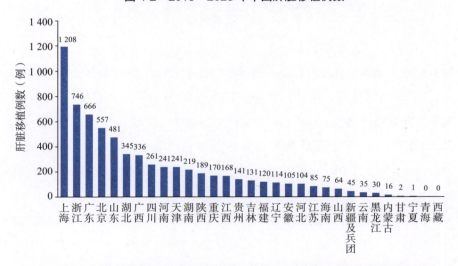

图 4-3　2023 年中国各省（自治区、直辖市）肝脏移植例数地区分布

2023年，共有110所医疗机构开展了肝脏移植，其中，有12所医疗机构实施的肝脏移植例数≥150例，其移植总量占全国当年总例数的42.9%；有10所医疗机构实施的肝脏移植例数在100~149例，其移植总量占全国当年总例数的17.9%；有21所医疗机构实施的肝脏移植例数在50~99例，其移植总量占全国当年总例数的20.8%；有27所医疗机构实施的肝脏移植例数在20~49例，其移植总量占全国当年总例数的14.1%；有40所医疗机构实施的肝脏移植例数<20例，其移植总量占全国当年总例数的4.3%。2023年中国实施肝脏移植例数排名前十位的医疗机构见表4-1。

表4-1 2023年中国肝脏移植例数排名前十位的医疗机构

地区	肝脏移植医疗机构	例数
上海	上海交通大学医学院附属仁济医院	583
浙江	浙江大学医学院附属第一医院	351
上海	复旦大学附属华山医院	280
天津	天津市第一中心医院	241
四川	四川大学华西医院	226
上海	复旦大学附属中山医院	206
山东	青岛大学附属医院	203
河南	郑州大学第一附属医院	199
浙江	树兰（杭州）医院	175
广西	广西医科大学第二附属医院	171

二、肝脏移植受体人口特征

2023年，中国肝脏移植受体的年龄均值为43.0岁，中位数49.8岁；受体体重指数(body mass index，BMI)均值22.4 kg/m^2，中位数22.5 kg/m^2；以男性受体为主，占比73.8%；受体血型以O型、A型、B型为主，且3种血型的受体各占约30%，血型为AB型的受体占比最少（表4-2）。

表 4-2　2023 年中国肝脏移植受体人口特征

变量	均值 ± 标准差	占比（%）	变量	占比（%）
年龄（岁）	43.0 ± 20.6	—	血型	
BMI（kg/m²）	22.4 ± 4.5	—	O 型	31.0
性别			A 型	30.7
男	—	73.8	B 型	28.0
女	—	26.2	AB 型	10.3

三、肝脏移植质量安全分析

1. 肝脏移植重要临床指标

2023 年，中国 LDLT 的平均冷缺血时间、平均无肝期、术中平均失血量、术中平均输红细胞量均低于 DDLT，LDLT 的平均手术时间略高于 DDLT。2015—2022 年和 2023 年这两个时段的重要临床指标均值对比情况见图 4-4 至图 4-8。

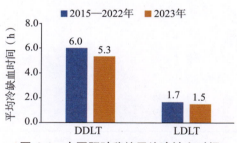

图 4-4　中国肝脏移植平均冷缺血时间

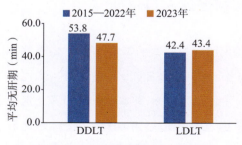

图 4-5　中国肝脏移植平均无肝期

第四章 中国肝脏移植

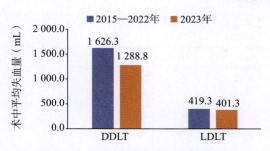

图 4-6　中国肝脏移植术中平均失血量

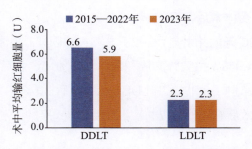

图 4-7　中国肝脏移植术中平均输红细胞量

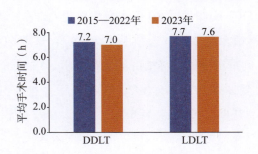

图 4-8　中国肝脏移植平均手术时间

2. 肝脏移植前后受体总胆红素的变化情况

分别对 2023 年 DDLT 受体和 LDLT 受体术前、术后各时间点的总胆红素变化情况进行分析，移植受体术后总胆红素平均值呈明显下降趋势（表 4-3）。

表 4-3 2023 年中国肝脏移植受体术前、术后的总胆红素平均值

单位：μmol/L

时间	DDLT	LDLT
术前	215.5	190.9
术后 1 周	68.0	48.3
术后 2 周	49.0	26.8
术后 1 月	32.5	18.1
术后 3 月	21.1	10.5
术后 6 月	20.8	9.7

3. 肝脏移植受体术后情况

（1）术后 30 天内并发症：2023 年，中国 DDLT 受体术后 30 天内并发症发生率为 24.0%，主要为胸腔积液（14.6%）、术后感染（9.3%）、腹腔积液/腹腔脓肿（8.9%）；LDLT 受体术后 30 天内并发症发生率为 21.0%，主要为术后感染（13.7%）、腹腔积液/腹腔脓肿（10.5%）、胸腔积液（9.7%）。

（2）术后 30 天内死亡率：2023 年，中国 DDLT 受体术后 30 天内死亡率为 4.9%；LDLT 受体术后 30 天内死亡率为 2.1%。

（3）肝脏移植术后受体、移植肝生存情况：选取 2015—2023 年开展的肝脏移植病例进行受体和移植肝的生存分析，结果如下。

中国 DDLT 受体术后 1 年、3 年、5 年累积生存率分别为 84.2%、74.9%、69.3%；LDLT 受体术后 1 年、3 年、5 年累积生存率分别为 93.6%、91.8%、91.3%。

中国 DDLT 移植肝术后 1 年、3 年、5 年累积生存率分别为 83.4%、73.9%、68.2%；LDLT 移植肝术后 1 年、3 年、5 年累积生存率分别为 92.9%、90.8%、90.0%（表 4-4）。

表 4-4 2015—2023 年中国肝脏移植受体/移植肝术后生存率

单位：%

分组	术后 1 年		术后 3 年		术后 5 年	
	受体	移植肝	受体	移植肝	受体	移植肝
DDLT	84.2	83.4	74.9	73.9	69.3	68.2
LDLT	93.6	92.9	91.8	90.8	91.3	90.0

（4）肝癌肝脏移植受体术后无瘤生存情况：2015—2023年，中国肝癌肝脏移植受体术后1年、3年、5年无瘤生存率分别为75.0%、61.0%、54.1%。

四、特点与展望

1. 肝脏移植例数创历史新高

在国家政策的有力引导、法律法规不断完善、整体医疗水平飞速提高的背景下，经过全国移植界专家学者的共同努力，我国肝脏移植规模稳步增长，移植质量与技术创新不断完善与提升。中国每年开展的肝脏移植例数稳居全球第二位，2023年，中国肝脏移植例数突破6 800例，年实施例数达到历年顶峰。

2. 受体年龄分布相对集中，中国儿童肝脏移植稳步发展

对比中国和美国2023年肝脏移植受体的年龄段分布，两国受体的年龄都主要集中在50～64岁，中国为41.9%，美国为44.5%。

随着中国儿童肝脏移植技术的日益成熟，其数量和移植质量也稳步发展，自2018年以来，中国儿童肝脏移植每年实施例数均达到1 000例以上。2023年，中国开展儿童肝脏移植1 209例，以6岁以下儿童肝脏移植为主，占儿童肝脏移植的80.4%；美国开展儿童肝脏移植534例，6岁以下儿童占儿童肝脏移植的62.5%。

3. 积极拓展供肝来源

LDLT和劈离式肝脏移植（split liver transplantation，SLT）是扩大供肝来源的重要途径，2023年有50余家移植中心开展了相关移植，开展规模地区差异较明显。实施LDLT前三位的省（自治区、直辖市）是上海（336例）、浙江（169例）、天津（119例），占全国LDLT的67.5%。开展SLT前三位的省（自治区、直辖市）是浙江（217例）、上海（75例）、广东（58例），占全国SLT的68.0%。

4. 持续推动肝脏移植精细化管理

在国家卫生健康委员会的领导下，围绕肝脏移植临床技术和术后管理水平、CLTR 系统数据填报情况进行飞行检查与调研工作；国家肝脏移植质控中心和 COTRS 联合组织开展全国肝脏移植超紧急状态（1A）病历核查工作；聚焦复杂肝移植、"肝癌肝移植 No-touch 新技术"等进行技术交流、推广与应用；围绕质控体系建设、规范和指南的制定与推广、肝脏移植技术培训、质控信息监测与反馈等方面有序开展工作，持续推动肝脏移植医疗质量和服务水平提升。

第五章 中国肾脏移植

数据范围介绍

本章内容主要基于中国肾脏移植科学登记系统（Chinese Scientific Registry of Kidney Transplantation，CSRKT），选取 2015 年 1 月 1 日至 2023 年 12 月 31 的数据分析。

统计方法介绍

对器官移植受体的基本情况采用描述性统计分析。

章节要点

（1）自 2015 年以来，本年度肾脏移植总例数创造历史新高：2023 年总例数较 2022 年（12 712 例）增长 17.7%，其中遗体器官捐献（deceased donor，DD）肾脏移植较 2022 年（10 187 例）增长 13.6%，亲属间活体（living-related donor，LD）肾脏移植较 2022 年（2 525 例）增长 34.4%。2023 年儿童肾脏移植例数继续回升，与 2021 年基本相当。2023 年肾脏相关多器官联合移植例数有突破性发展，较 2022 年增长 36.5%。2023 年有 6 所医疗机构实施共 7 例单独的胰腺移植。

（2）肾脏移植例数的分布依然呈现地区优势和大型移植中心优势：2023 年有 10 个省（自治区、直辖市）实施肾脏移植≥600 例，其移植例数占全国总例数的 68.2%；实施肾脏移植例数＞250 例的医疗机构有 14 所，其移植例数占全国总例数的 38.2%。

（3）大部分肾脏移植受体为男性，2023 年肾脏移植男性受体占

69.2%。

（4）肾脏移植术后总体生存率满意，但需加强肾脏移植相关的多器官联合移植受体管理：2023年数据显示肾脏移植术后1年、3年、5年总体生存率满意，但胰肾联合移植的术后感染率较高，且受体死亡导致的移植物丢失占比过高。

一、肾脏移植医疗机构分布

截至2023年底，共有149所医疗机构具备肾脏移植资质，医疗机构数量排名前十位的省（自治区、直辖市）为广东（18所）、北京（13所）、湖南（10所）、山东（10所）、浙江（9所）、上海（8所）、湖北（7所）、广西（6所）、河南（6所）和江苏（6所）（图5-1）。

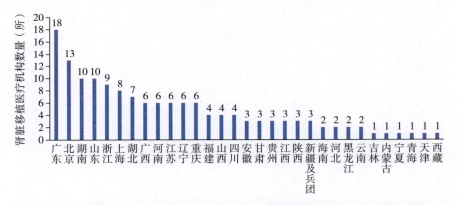

图5-1　2023年中国各省（自治区、直辖市）具有肾脏移植资质的医疗机构地区分布

2015—2023年，中国共实施肾脏移植102 761例，其中DD肾脏移植83 624例，LD肾脏移植19 137例。2023年，中国共实施肾脏移植14 968例，较2022年增长17.7%，其中DD肾脏移植11 575例，较2022年增长13.6%；LD肾脏移植3 393例，较2022年增长34.4%（图5-2）。

2023年中国实施肾脏移植例数排名前十位的省（自治区、直辖市）依次为广东（1 626例）、山东（1 335例）、湖北（1 104例）、河南（1 026例）、广西（955例）、北京（906例）、四川（877例）、浙江

（849例）、湖南（791例）和上海（732例）。各省（自治区、直辖市）实施的肾脏移植例数见图5-3。

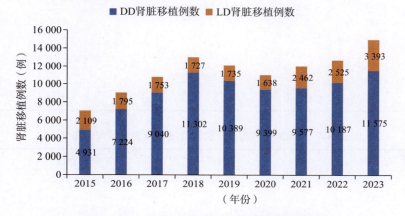

图5-2　2015—2023年中国肾脏移植例数

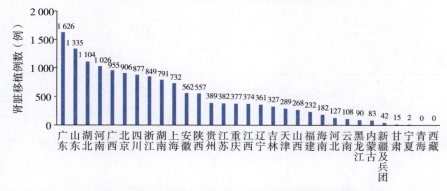

图5-3　2023年中国各省（自治区、直辖市）肾脏移植例数地区分布

2023年中国肾脏移植手术的开展具有地区优势，有10个省实施肾脏移植≥600例，占全国总例数的68.2%（表5-1）。

2023年实施肾脏移植≥250例的医疗机构有14所，其移植例数占总例数的38.2%；另外，200~249例的有6所，100~199例的有35所，50~99例的有27所，10~49例的有39所，1~9例的有13所。此外，有15所未开展肾脏移植，其中12所连续3年未开展肾脏移植（表5-2）。

表 5-1　2023 年中国各省（自治区、直辖市）肾脏移植例数分布

例数区间	省（区、市）数	例数占比（%）
≥ 600	10	68.2
400～599	2	7.5
200～399	9	20
100～199	3	2.8
1～99	5	1.5
0	2	0

表 5-2　2023 年中国医疗机构肾脏移植例数区间分布

例数区间	医疗机构数	例数占比（%）
≥ 250	14	38.2
200～249	6	9.0
100～199	35	31.6
50～99	27	13.0
10～49	39	7.7
1～9	13	0.4
0	15	0

2023 年，中国 DD 肾脏移植例数排名前十位的省（自治区、直辖市）为广东、山东、广西、湖北、北京、河南、湖南、上海、浙江和陕西，其例数占 DD 总例数的 69.3%（图 5-4），排名前十位的医疗机构见表 5-3。

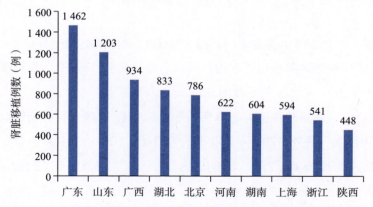

图 5-4　2023 年中国 DD 肾脏移植例数前十位的省（自治区、直辖市）

表 5-3　2023 年中国 DD 肾脏移植例数排名前十位的医疗机构

地区	肾脏移植医疗机构	DD 例数	总例数
广西	广西医科大学第二附属医院	416	419
陕西	西安交通大学第一附属医院	403	504
河南	郑州大学第一附属医院	368	569
上海	上海交通大学医学院附属仁济医院	362	439
四川	四川大学华西医院	314	711
广东	中山大学附属第一医院	305	348
浙江	浙江大学医学院附属第一医院	295	560
山东	青岛大学附属医院	257	267
湖北	华中科技大学同济医学院附属同济医院	253	418
山东	山东省千佛山医院	252	276

2023 年中国 LD 肾脏移植例数排名前十位的省为四川、河南、安徽、浙江、湖北、天津、湖南、广东、上海和山东（图 5-5），排名前十位的医疗机构见表 5-4。

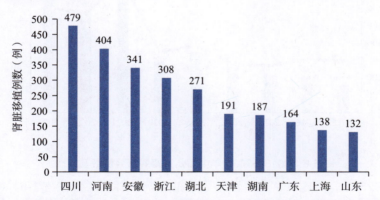

图 5-5　2023 年中国 LD 肾脏移植例数排名前十位的省（自治区、直辖市）

表 5-4　2023 年中国 LD 肾脏移植例数排名前十位的医疗机构

地区	肾脏移植医疗机构	LD 例数	总例数
四川	四川大学华西医院	397	711
浙江	浙江大学医学院附属第一医院	265	560
安徽	中国科学技术大学附属第一医院	236	325

续表

地区	肾脏移植医疗机构	LD 例数	总例数
河南	郑州大学第一附属医院	201	569
天津	天津市第一中心医院	191	289
湖北	华中科技大学同济医学院附属同济医院	165	418
湖南	中南大学湘雅二医院	132	267
河南	河南省人民医院	118	159
陕西	西安交通大学第一附属医院	101	504
安徽	安徽医科大学第一附属医院	100	194

2023 年，中国共实施儿童肾脏移植（<18 岁）669 例，占全国当年总例数的 4.5%，较 2022 年增长 16.3%（图 5-6）。其中，受体<1 岁 2 例、1~<6 岁 46 例、6~<14 岁 283 例、14~<18 岁 338 例。

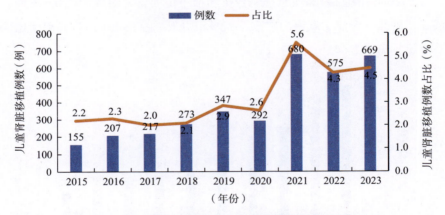

图 5-6　2015—2023 年中国儿童肾脏移植例数及占比

2023 年，中国共实施单独胰腺移植 7 例，肝胰联合移植 1 例，肾脏相关多器官联合移植 116 例，较 2022 年（85 例）增长 36.5%，其中肝肾联合移植 42 例、胰肾联合移植 68 例、心肾联合移植 6 例（图 5-7）。2023 年各省（自治区、直辖市）实施肾脏相关多器官联合移植例数见图 5-8。2023 年实施单独胰腺移植的医疗机构见表 5-5，肾脏相关多器官联合移植例数排名前十位的医疗机构见表 5-6。

第五章　中国肾脏移植

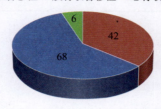

图 5-7　2023 年中国肾脏相关多器官联合移植实施例数

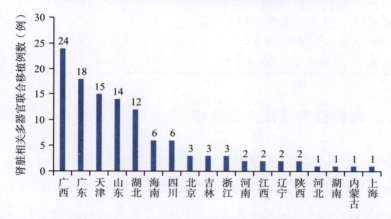

图 5-8　2023 年中国各省（自治区、直辖市）实施肾脏相关多器官联合移植例数

表 5-5　2023 年中国实施单独胰腺移植的医疗机构

地区	肾脏移植医疗机构	例数
四川	四川省人民医院	2
山西	山西白求恩医院	1
山东	山东省千佛山医院	1
山东	青岛大学附属医院	1
辽宁	中国医科大学附属第一医院	1
湖北	华中科技大学同济医学院附属同济医院	1

表 5-6　2023 年中国肾脏相关多器官联合移植例数排名前十位的医疗机构

地区	肾脏移植医疗机构	例数
广西	广西医科大学第二附属医院	21
天津	天津市第一中心医院	15

47

续表

地区	肾脏移植医疗机构	例数
湖北	华中科技大学同济医学院附属同济医院	12
广东	中山大学附属第一医院	9
山东	青岛大学附属医院	8
海南	海南医学院第二附属医院	5
山东	山东省千佛山医院	5
广东	广州医科大学附属第二医院	4
四川	四川省人民医院	4
吉林	吉林大学白求恩第一医院	3

二、肾脏移植受体人口特征

2023年，中国肾脏移植受体年龄（40.2±12.5）岁，BMI（22.1±3.6）kg/m^2，术前中位透析时间662天，男性受体占69.2%，O血型受体最多，占33.3%，AB血型受体最少，占9.8%（表5–7）。

表5-7 2023年中国肾脏移植受体人口特征

变量	均值 ± 标准差
受体年龄（岁）	40.2 ± 12.5
BMI（kg/m^2）	22.1 ± 3.6
透析时间	中位数（四分位间距）
术前透析时间（天）	662（304 ~ 1 248）
受体血型	数量（占比，%）
O 型	4 977（33.3）
A 型	4 395（29.4）
B 型	4 123（27.5）
AB 型	1 473（9.8）
性别	例数（占比，%）
男	10 362（69.2）
女	4 606（30.8）

受体年龄区间分布为儿童（＜18岁）受体677例，占比4.5%；18～＜30岁的受体2 139例，占14.3%；30～＜50岁的受体8 349例，占55.8%；50～＜65岁受体3 545例，占23.7%；老年（≥65岁）受体266例，占1.8%。

三、肾脏移植质量安全分析

1. 供肾缺血时间

分别对2023年LD、DD肾脏移植病例进行分析，供肾平均冷缺血时间、热缺血时间均在标准范围内（表5-8）。

表5-8　2023年LD、DD肾脏移植供肾缺血时间

变量	LD（均值±标准差）	DD（均值±标准差）
供肾冷缺血时间/h	2.1±1.6	5.8±3.9
供肾热缺血时间/min	3.0±2.0	5.1±3.7

2023年，LD肾脏移植和DD肾脏移植中，供肾冷缺血时间≤24小时占比分别为99.7%和98.9%；热缺血时间≤10分钟的占比分别为98.6%和72.7%，2023年DD肾脏移植有27.3%的移植受体热缺血时间＞10分钟（表5-9）。

表5-9　2023年LD、DD肾脏移植供肾缺血时间占比

变量	LD（%）	DD（%）
供肾冷缺血时间≤24 h	99.7	98.9
供肾热缺血时间≤10 min	98.6	72.7

2. 肾脏移植手术前后受体血清肌酐值的变化情况

对2023年肾脏移植手术病例术前、术后30天、术后180天和术后360天4个时间点的血清肌酐进行分析，LD与DD肾脏移植受体的血清肌酐平均值见表5-10。对2015—2023年的病例进行分析，LD和DD肾脏移植术前及术后各时间点的血清肌酐平均值分别为术前996.5 μmol/L、941.3 μmol/L，

术后 30 天 125.7 μmol/L、151.6 μmol/L，术后 180 天 120.6 μmol/L、128.6 μmol/L，术后 360 天 97.3 μmol/L、118.2 μmol/L。

表 5-10　2023 年 LD、DD 肾脏移植受体术前、术后的血清肌酐平均值

时间点	LD（μmol/L）	DD（μmol/L）
术前	996.5	941.3
术后 30 天	125.7	151.6
术后 180 天	120.6	128.6
术后 360 天	97.3	118.2

3. 肾脏移植术后不良事件概况

肾脏移植术后不良事件主要包括移植肾功能延迟恢复、急性排异反应、感染、移植肾全因丢失、移植受体死亡等。对 2023 年病例的随访资料进行分析，主要不良事件发生率见表 5-11。受体术后 30 天内死亡率为 0.3%。对 2023 年肾脏相关多器官联合移植病例进行分析，主要不良事件发生率见表 5-12。

表 5-11　2023 年中国肾脏移植术后不良事件发生率

不良事件	LD（%）	DD（%）
移植肾功能延迟恢复	1.9	14.9
急性排异反应	1.7	3.3
感染	4.0	7.7
移植肾全因丢失	1.6	4.4
移植受体死亡	0.2	1.2

表 5-12　2023 年中国肾脏相关多器官联合移植术后不良事件发生率

不良事件	发生率（%）
移植肾功能延迟恢复	7.8
急性排异反应	2.6
感染	9.6
移植肾全因丢失	10.4
移植受体死亡	6.1

4. 肾脏移植受体、移植物生存分析

对 2015—2023 年中国开展的 102 761 例肾脏移植受体/移植物（以下简称"人/肾"）进行生存分析，采用 Kaplan-meier 法计算累积生存率。LD 肾脏移植的 1 年人/肾生存率为 99.1%/98.4%，DD 肾脏移植的 1 年人/肾生存率为 97.5%/95.5%；LD 肾脏移植的 3 年人/肾生存率为 98.5%/96.3%，DD 肾脏移植的 3 年人/肾生存率为 96.2%/92.6%；LD 肾脏移植的 5 年人/肾生存率为 97.8%/93.1%，DD 肾脏移植的 5 年人/肾生存率为 94.7%/88.8%（表 5-13）。

表 5-13 2015—2023 年中国肾脏移植受体/移植肾术后生存率

单位：%

供体类别	术后 1 年		术后 3 年		术后 5 年	
	受体	移植肾	受体	移植肾	受体	移植肾
LD 肾脏	99.1	98.4	98.5	96.3	97.8	93.1
DD 肾脏	97.5	95.5	96.2	92.6	94.7	88.8

四、特点与展望

1. 肾脏移植总例数创历史新高，LD 肾脏移植例数增长显著

2023 年，中国肾脏移植数量创历史新高，总例数较 2022 年（12 712 例）增长 17.7%。其中，LD 肾脏移植增长明显，总例数达 3 393 例，为历年之最，较 2022 年增长 34.4%。移植例数的显著增长不仅反映我国在遗体捐献工作体系和管理机制方面的日趋成熟，也提示基于 LD 肾脏移植的良好预后，这可能与较多移植中心进一步优化了亲属间活体器官捐献的流程，提高了工作效率有关。

2. 儿童肾脏移植例数回升

儿童肾脏移植例数近年来持续上升，2023 年例数（669 例）较 2022 年增长 16.3%，其中 LD 肾脏移植 45 例（6.7%），DD 肾脏移植 624 例（93.3%）。在年龄分布上，≤14 岁的受体 331 例（48.4%），有 589 名

（88.0%）接受了儿童捐献的肾脏，其中＜1岁的儿童供肾37例（5.5%），提示低龄/低体重儿童供肾的肾脏移植逐渐在临床开展，如何在器官捐献及移植手术管理方面进行优质、高效地利用低龄/低体重儿童供肾，是值得探讨的重要话题。

3. 肾脏移植在例数分布上继续呈地区和大型移植中心优势

2023年，肾脏移植例数排名前十位的省（自治区、直辖市）分别为广东、山东、湖北、河南、广西、北京、四川、浙江、湖南和上海，占全国当年总例数的68.2%，地区优势明显。2023年实施肾脏移植≥250例的医疗机构有14所，较2022年增加4所，其实施肾脏移植例数占全国肾脏移植总例数的38.2%；≥100例的医疗机构55所，其实施肾脏移植例数占全国总例数的78.8%，此外还有1所医疗机构突破了700例，大型移植中心例数优势十分明显。

4. 关注多器官联合移植

2023年，肾脏相关多器官联合移植例数较2022年增长了36.5%，有7所医疗机构实施了7例单独胰腺移植。与单独肾脏移植相比，胰肾联合移植术后不良事件尤其是移植肾全因丢失和受体死亡发生率相对较高。

5. 关注肾脏移植研究热点，更新临床指南

为进一步推动肾脏移植临床诊疗的同质化管理，提高肾脏移植医疗服务质量，多项临床指南正在撰写或修订中。此外，针对肾脏捐献及移植工作中新凸显的问题例如低龄/低体重儿童供肾的合理分配与利用、胰腺移植和胰肾联合移植的科学管理等，我国专家学者正在探索并制定适合本国国情的共识与指南。

第六章 中国心脏移植

数据范围介绍

心脏移植章节内容数据来源于中国心脏移植注册系统（China Heart Transplant Registry，CHTR），选取2015年1月1日至2023年12月31日的数据。

统计方法介绍

对心脏移植手术数据的基本情况采用描述性统计分析，采用生存分析法计算累积生存率。

章节要点

（1）近年来，中国心脏移植例数逐年增加，2023年为994例，较2022年提升40%，全国共76家心脏移植资质医院，分布在29个省份，医疗可及性逐年扩大。

（2）心脏移植术前心肺运动试验检查率、供体心脏缺血时间和术后院内结局等质量指标持续改善。

（3）心脏移植术后30天、术后1年、术后3年和术后5年生存率分别为93.1%、81.5%、76.1%和70.2%，达到国际水平。

一、心脏移植医疗机构分布

截至2023底，中国共有76所医疗机构具备心脏移植资质，其中，心脏移植医疗机构数量较多的省（自治区、直辖市）依次为广东（8所）、浙江（7所）、北京（5所）、上海（5所）和湖北（5所）（图6-1）。

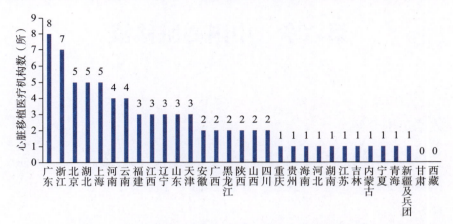

图6-1　2023年中国各省（自治区、直辖市）心脏移植医疗机构分布

2015—2023年，中国共实施心脏移植手术共5 261例（图6-2）。2023年开展心脏移植手术994例，较2022年提升40%，其中儿童（＜18岁）心脏移植125例，占总例数的12.6%，心肺联合移植2例。各省（自治区、直辖市）心脏移植例数分布见图6-3。

2023年，全国共64所医疗机构开展心脏移植手术，其中2所医疗机构例数≥100例，2所医疗机构例数≥50例（图6-4）。2023年中国心脏移植例数排名前十位的医疗机构见图6-5。

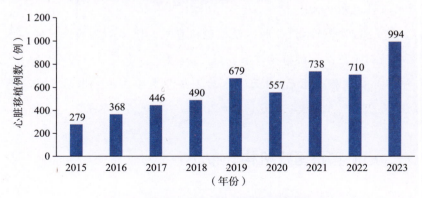

图6-2　2015—2023年中国心脏移植例数

第六章 中国心脏移植

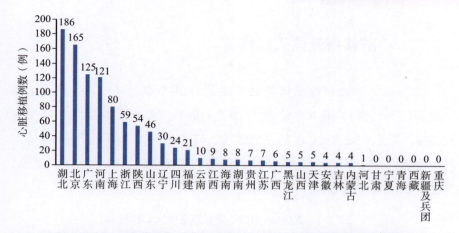

图 6-3 2023 年中国各省（自治区、直辖市）心脏移植例数分布情况

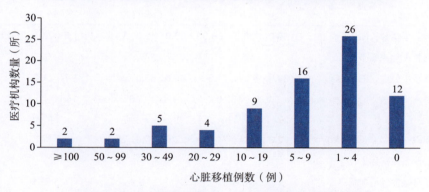

图 6-4 2023 年中国医疗机构心脏移植例数区间分布情况

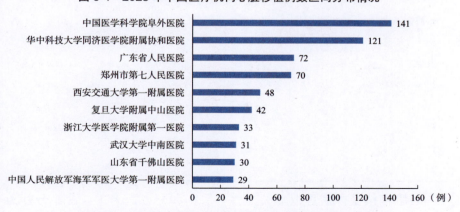

图 6-5 2023 年中国心脏移植例数排名前十位的医疗机构

二、心脏移植受体人口特征

2023 年，心脏移植受体年龄中位数为 50.0 岁，其中，男性受体比例为 76.7%；受体 BMI 中位数为 22.2 kg/m^2。移植受体血型中 O 型占 28.0%，A 型占 33.0%，B 型占 29.2%，AB 型占 9.9%。成人移植受体年龄中位数为 53.0 岁，男性占 78.8%；儿童移植受体年龄中位数为 11.0 岁，男性占 63.2%（表 6-1）。

表 6-1　2023 年中国心脏移植受体人口特征

变量	总体移植受体（n=994）	成人移植受体（n=869）	儿童移植受体（n=125）
年龄中位数，IQR（岁）	50.0（34.0, 58.0）	53.0（42.0, 59.0）	11.0（7.0, 14.0）
男性占比（%）	76.7	78.8	63.2
体重中位数，IQR（kg）	64.0（51.7, 71.6）	65.0（56.0, 73.0）	33.7（21.0, 47.5）
身高中位数，IQR（cm）	168.5（160.0, 173.0）	170.0（163.0, 174.0）	145.0（127.0, 165.0）
BMI 中位数，IQR（kg/m^2）	22.2（19.1, 24.7）	22.6（20.2, 25.1）	15.6（13.2, 19.7）
心脏移植病因占比（%）			
非缺血性心肌病	76.8	75.8	83.5
冠心病	12.6	14.4	0.8
心脏瓣膜病	3.1	3.4	1.5
先天性心脏病	2.2	1.3	8.3
其他疾病	5.3	5.1	5.9
ABO 血型占比（%）			
A	33.0	33.5	29.6
B	29.2	30.1	22.4
O	28.0	26.1	30.8
AB	9.9	10.3	7.2

心脏移植受体病因以非缺血性心肌病和冠心病为主，占比分别为 76.8% 和 12.6%，其次为心脏瓣膜病（3.1%）和先天性心脏病（2.2%）。

成人受体病因以非缺血性心肌病（75.8%）和冠心病（14.4%）为主；儿童受体病因以非缺血性心肌病（83.5%）和先天性心脏病（8.3%）为主。

三、心脏移植质量安全分析

1. 术前心肺运动试验检查率

心肺运动试验是判断患者是否符合心脏移植适应证的首选方法。对于不存在心肺运动试验禁忌证的移植候选患者，采用该试验进行心脏移植入选评估，能够帮助医生了解移植受体心脏以外器官功能状况是否正常，并及时纠正存在的问题。

2023年我国成人心脏移植接受术前心肺运动试验的检查率为57.2%，比2022年提升12.8%（表6-2）。

表6-2　2022年和2023年中国心脏移植术前心肺运动试验检查率

年份	术前心肺运动试验检查率（%）
2022年	44.4
2023年	57.2

2. 供体心脏缺血时间

供体心脏缺血时间是指供体心脏获取直至植入受体体内之间的时间。研究表明供体心脏保存技术通常允许≤6 h的安全缺血时间。供体心脏的缺血时间≤6 h的占比是反映医疗机构供体心脏选择和维护规范性的重要指标。

2023年，心脏移植供体心脏缺血时间中位数为3.3 h，与2022年供体缺血时间中位数相比下降0.3 h（表6-3），心脏移植供体缺血时间≤6 h的移植患者占比为85.3%。

表6-3　2022年和2023年中国心脏移植供体缺血时间情况

年份	供体缺血时间，IQR（h）	供体缺血时间≤6小时占比（%）
2022年	3.6（2.5，5.5）	88.0
2023年	3.3（2.3，5.3）	85.3

3. 术后院内生存情况

2023年，中国心脏移植受体院内存活率为94.2%。心脏移植受体术后感染发生率为16.7%，其他术后主要并发症分别为心脏骤停（3.8%）、二次开胸（4.6%）、气管切开（5.1%）和二次插管（9.6%）。心脏移植受体院内主要死亡原因中，多器官功能衰竭占11.3%，移植心脏衰竭和感染分别占6.5%和32.3%（表6-4）。

表6-4 2023年心脏移植受体术后院内生存情况

变量	构成比（%）		
	总体（n=994）	成人移植受体（n=869）	儿童移植受体（n=125）
院内存活	94.2	93.6	97.7
术后并发症			
术后感染	16.7	16.9	9.8
心脏骤停	3.8	6.8	8.3
二次开胸	4.6	6.5	9.8
气管切开	5.1	6.7	9.8
二次插管	9.6	6.5	8.3
院内死亡原因			
多器官功能衰竭	11.3	11.9	0
移植心脏衰竭	6.5	6.8	0
感染	32.3	33.9	0
脑血管原因	27.4	23.7	100
急性排异	6.5	6.8	0
其他	16	16.9	0

4. 生存分析

2015—2023年，中国心脏移植术后30天、术后1年、术后3年和术后5年的生存率分别为93.1%、81.5%、76.1%和70.2%。其中，成人心脏移植术后30天、术后1年、术后3年和术后5年生存率分别为92.2%、80.8%、75.6%和70.6%；儿童心脏移植术后30天、术后1年、术后3年和术后5年生存率分别为94.8%、87.2%、81.6%和73.3%（表6-5）。

表 6-5　2015—2023 年心脏移植术后生存率

单位：%

	术后 30 天	术后 1 年	术后 3 年	术后 5 年
总体移植受体	93.1	81.5	76.1	70.2
成人移植受体	92.2	80.8	75.6	70.6
儿童移植受体	94.8	87.2	81.6	73.3

四、特点与展望

1. 心脏移植例数逐年增加，医疗机构间差异明显

近年来，我国心脏移植发展迅速，心脏移植例数逐年上升，2023 年共完成心脏移植 994 例，比 2022 年增长 40%。除西藏和甘肃外，各省（自治区、直辖市）均具有心脏移植医疗机构，为广大患者提供了较高的心脏移植医疗可及性。

中国医学科学院阜外医院和华中科技大学同济医学院附属协和医院年均心脏移植例数 > 100 例，单中心移植规模和质量达到世界领先水平；广东省人民医院、复旦大学附属中山医院、郑州市第七人民医院等医疗机构年均例数保持在 50 例左右，具备较为稳定的心脏移植服务能力。但医疗机构间技术能力仍然存在较大差异，2023 年全国有 12 家医疗机构未开展心脏移植手术，42 家医疗机构心脏移植手术例数 < 10 例；以上医疗机构具备心脏移植资质但未能有效提供或开展心脏移植临床服务。

为此，制定医疗机构间对口帮扶计划，推广优秀医疗机构的心脏移植管理经验和发展理念，将是下一步全国心脏移植质量提升工作的重点。

2. 心脏供体短缺仍然是限制心脏移植例数增长的重要因素

目前我国心脏移植例数的增长仍然受到供体器官匮乏的限制，COTRS 数据显示，2023 年我国每捐献者获取心脏数为 0.16，低于发达国家水平。2020—2023 年，我国脑死亡来源器官捐献者的占比大幅度提高，2023 年达到 70.7%，这为提高心脏捐献率提供了较大空间。

为此，2024 年，国家心脏移植医疗质控中心将联合国家人体捐献器官获取质控中心和国家卫生健康委人体组织器官移植与医疗大数据中心，在全国范围内开展心脏捐献供体源头培训，提高 OPO 和移植医院的供体评估、维护和获取能力，提高心脏供体捐献率和捐献质量。

3. 进一步加强心脏移植医师培训和团队建设

中国心脏移植的快速发展离不开各家医疗机构移植医师团队的有力支撑，但目前我国心脏移植外科医师的数量仍然不能满足日益增加的手术需求，2023 年具备心脏移植资质的医疗机构平均心脏移植外科医师为 3.1 名，其中仅有 85 名心脏移植医师开展了心脏移植手术。此外，心脏移植内科医师的培训和认证需要得到重视，目前我国现有的心脏移植医师资质认证规范仅限于外科医师，而心脏移植的诊疗过程，包括心脏移植术前评估、术后康复和远期随访等重要环节，都需要内科医师的高度参与。

因此，需要进一步重视心脏移植内科和外科医师技术能力培训和移植团队培训，制定相关的培训规范和制度，同时应当对未能开展心脏移植的医疗机构团队进行再次培训。

4. 持续推进心脏移植质量改进行动

从 2021 年开始，国家心脏移植质控中心通过发布技术规范和开展相关培训，聚焦全国各家医疗机构的移植质量提升工作，其中以提升术前心肺运动试验检查率的质量改进行动为代表，术前检查率从 2022 年的 44.4% 提升到 2023 年的 57.2%，持续优化心脏移植术前评估和受体筛选环节。

2024 年，心脏移植质控中心将持续推进心脏移植重点环节的质量改进行动，重点开展心脏移植术后并发症治疗以及术后随访的质量核查和改善工作，同时制订中国心脏移植临床指南，进一步推动心脏移植临床诊疗的同质化发展。

第七章 中国肺脏移植

数据范围介绍

中国肺脏移植章节内容数据来源于中国肺脏移植注册系统（China Lung Transplantation Registry，CLuTR），选取2015年1月1日至2023年12月31日的数据。

统计方法介绍

对中国肺脏移植的基本情况采用描述性统计分析，累积生存率采用Kaplan-Meier法统计。

章节要点

（1）2023年，中国共完成肺脏移植手术959例，其中单肺移植361例（37.6%），双肺移植596例（62.2%），心肺联合移植2例（0.2%）；中国成人肺脏移植男性受体占85.1%，年龄为（42.3±12.8）岁。移植数量前6所医疗机构的肺脏移植例数占总例数的69.5%，因此，应采取措施进一步促进医疗机构肺脏移植同质化发展。

（2）2023年，肺脏移植后受者30天存活率达到83.8%，气道吻合口并发症发生率、移植后急性排异反应发生率均有所下降，但原发性移植物失功发生率、围手术期感染发生率有所上升，需进一步加强质控指标的监测和动态反馈，持续推进全程化、多环节的并发症预防及控制工作机制。

（3）2023年，中国完成儿童肺脏移植22例，其中浙江大学医学院附属第二医院完成14例，无锡市人民医院完成6例；中国儿童肺脏移植男性受体占63.6%，年龄为（12.5±3.5）岁。术后30天存活率≥90%，提示儿童肺脏移植技术正在逐渐完善，走向成熟，亟须制订适合我国国情的儿童肺脏移植行业技术性指导文件，以促进儿童肺脏移植技术的长足发展，改善长期预后。

一、肺脏移植医疗机构分布

截至2023年底，中国共有60所医疗机构取得肺脏移植资质，覆盖全国24个省（自治区、直辖市）。中国各省（自治区、直辖市）具有肺脏移植资质的医疗机构数量见图7-1。

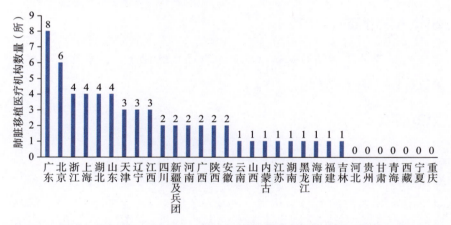

图7-1 2023年中国各省（自治区、直辖市）具有肺脏移植资质的医疗机构地区分布

2015—2023年，CLuTR共上报肺脏移植手术4 558例，各年度开展肺脏移植手术分别为118例、204例、299例、403例、489例、513例、775例、798例和959例（图7-2），呈逐年上升趋势。其中共上报儿童肺脏移植手术69例，各年度开展儿童肺脏移植手术分别为2例、1例、0例、3例、9例、8例、12例、12例、22例（图7-3）。

2023年，有43家医疗机构开展了肺脏移植手术。移植例数10例及以上的医疗机构见图7-4。2023年开展的22例儿童肺脏移植中，浙江大

第七章 中国肺脏移植

学医学院附属第二医院完成14例，无锡市人民医院完成6例，中国人民解放军总医院和中日友好医院各完成1例。

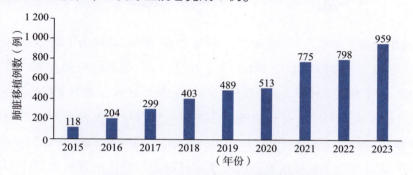

图7-2　2015—2023年中国肺脏移植例数

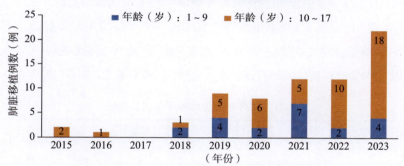

图7-3　2015—2023年中国儿童肺脏移植例数

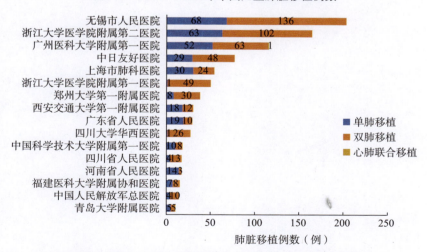

图7-4　2023年实施肺脏移植例数≥10例的医疗机构排名

二、肺脏移植受体人口特征

2023年中国成人肺脏移植男性受体占85.1%；年龄为（42.3±12.8）岁，＞60岁占47.8%。O型、A型、B型及AB型血型分别占33.5%、29.1%、26.7%及10.7%。移植前15.9%的受体在重症监护室（Intensive Care Unit，ICU）住院；心功能状态方面，日常活动完全受限纽约心脏病学会功能分级（New York Heart Association Functional Classification，NYHA功能分级）Ⅳ级以及病情严重需住院治疗的比例分别为20.3%和21.6%。2023年中国儿童肺脏移植男性受体占63.6%；年龄为（12.5±3.5）岁。O型、A型、B型及AB型血型分别占50.0%、36.4%、9.1%及4.5%。移植前13.6%的受体在ICU住院；心功能状态方面，日常活动完全受限（NYHA Ⅳ级）以及病情严重需住院治疗的比例分别为13.6%和27.3%（表7-1）。

表7-1 2023年肺脏移植受体人口特征

变量（成人）	占比（%）	变量（儿童）	占比（%）
性别		性别	
男	85.1	男	63.6
女	14.9	女	36.4
年龄（岁）		年龄（岁）	
18～35	7.0	1～9	18.2
36～49	14.0	10～17	81.8
50～59	31.2	—	—
60～64	16.5	—	—
65～74	29.8	—	—
≥75	1.5	—	—
血型		血型	
O型	33.5	O型	50.0
A型	29.1	A型	36.4
B型	26.7	B型	9.1
AB型	10.7	AB型	4.5

续表

变量（成人）	占比（%）	变量（儿童）	占比（%）
移植前住院情况		移植前住院情况	
ICU	15.9	ICU	13.6
普通住院	69.7	普通住院	77.3
未住院	14.4	未住院	9.1
移植前心功能状态		移植前心功能状态	
无活动限制（NYHA I/II）	1.4	无活动限制（NYHA I/II）	0.0
日常活动部分受限（NYHA III）	56.7	日常活动部分受限（NYHA III）	59.1
日常活动完全受限（NYHA IV）	20.3	日常活动完全受限（NYHA IV）	13.6
病情严重需住院治疗	21.6	病情严重需住院治疗	27.3

2023年，中国成人肺脏移植受体原发病中，以特发性肺间质纤维化、慢性阻塞性肺疾病、继发性肺间质纤维化和肺尘埃沉着病为主，分别占37.6%、19.6%、11.7%和11.6%。此外，肺脏移植术后再移植、支气管扩张症、闭塞性细支气管炎、肺动脉高压和淋巴管平滑肌瘤病分别占4.1%、3.4%、2.8%、1.2%和0.3%（图7-5）。特发性肺间质纤维化、慢性阻塞性肺疾病、继发性肺间质纤维化和肺尘埃沉着病中，双肺脏移植比例分别为57.9%、61.9%、70.9%和37.6%。

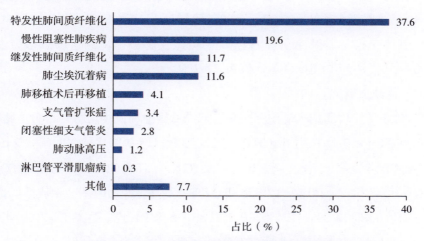

图7-5　2023年中国成人肺脏移植受体原发病分布

2023年，中国儿童肺脏移植受体原发病主要为闭塞性细支气管炎（13例），囊性纤维化、肺动静脉瘘、原发性肺动脉高压、继发性肺间质纤维化、继发性肺动脉高压患者，分别为3例、2例、2例、1例、1例（图7-6）。

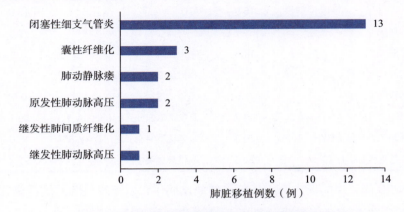

图7-6　2023年中国儿童肺脏移植受体原发病分布

三、肺脏移植质量安全分析

1. 手术方式

2023年，中国成人肺脏移植术中单、双肺脏移植分别占38.5%和61.3%，心肺联合移植占0.2%。急诊肺脏移植占14.2%，术中使用ECMO的比例为79.7%。儿童肺脏移植术中均为双肺移植，急诊肺脏移植占13.6%，术中使用ECMO的比例为77.3%。

2. 冷缺血时间

2023年，中国成人肺脏移植单、双肺冷缺血时间中位数（四分位距）分别为6.0（4.0～7.1）h和8.0（7.0～9.5）h。单肺冷缺血时间＜2 h、2～＜4 h、4～＜6 h、6～＜8 h、8～＜10 h、≥10 h的比例分别为1.5%、16.2%、27.2%、42.0%、12.5%和0.6%；双肺冷缺血时间在相应区间比例分别为0.4%、3.0%、12.4%、26.6%、35.7%和21.9%（图7-7）。2023年，中国儿童肺脏移植冷缺血时间中位数（四分位距）为8.0（7.5～9.0）h。

第七章 中国肺脏移植

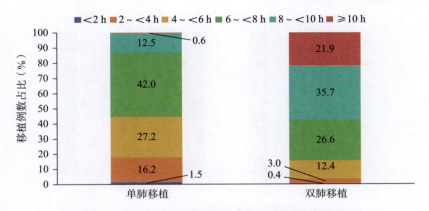

图 7-7　2023 年中国成人肺脏移植单、双肺冷缺血时间

3. 术中输血

术中成人受体输血量的中位数（四分位距）为 800.0（0.0～1 600.0）mL，＜500 mL、500～＜1 000 mL、1 000～＜1 500 mL、1 500～＜2 000 和 ≥2 000 mL 的比例分别为 39.7%、17.3%、14.8%、9.5% 和 18.7%。术中儿童受体输血量的中位数（四分位距）为 650.0（312.5～2 015.0）mL。

4. 术后并发症情况

2023 年，中国肺脏移植受体术后出院前移植物失功发生率为 15.7%，感染发生率为 66.6%，急性排异反应发生率为 3.3%，气道吻合口并发症发生率为 8.8%。2019—2023 年术后出院前移植物失功发生率见图 7-8，感染发生率见图 7-9，急性排异反应发生率见图 7-10，气道吻合口并发症发生率见图 7-11。

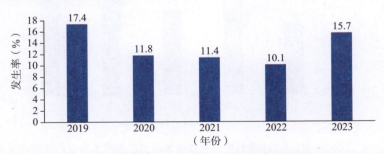

图 7-8　2019—2023 年中国肺脏移植受体术后出院前移植物失功发生率

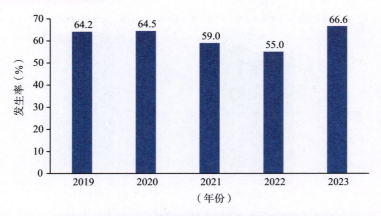

图 7-9　2019—2023 年中国肺脏移植受体术后出院前感染发生率

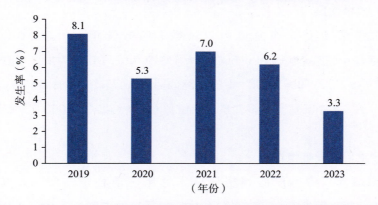

图 7-10　2019—2023 年中国肺脏移植受体术后出院前急性排异反应发生率

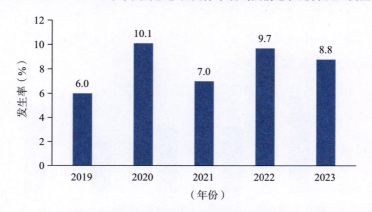

图 7-11　2019—2023 年中国肺脏移植受体术后出院前气道吻合口并发症发生率

第七章　中国肺脏移植

5. 出院时状态

2023年，中国成人肺脏移植受体ICU停留时间中位数（四分位距）为144.0（72.0～336.0）h；住院时间中位数（四分位距）为32.0（20.0～49.0）天；中国儿童肺脏移植受体ICU停留时间中位数（四分位距）为132.0（87.5～300.5）h；住院时间中位数（四分位距）为35.0（30.75～56.0）天。成人受体术后30天存活率为83.6%，30天内死因主要为多器官功能衰竭（29.4%）、感染（17.5%）、失血性休克（11.1%）和移植物失功（6.3%）（图7-12）。两例儿童在术后30天内死亡的原因分别为多器官功能衰竭和吻合口并发症。

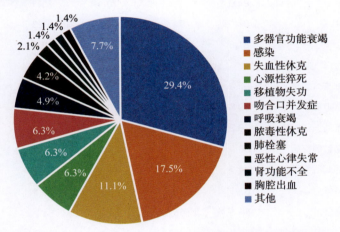

图7-12　2023年中国成人肺脏移植受体术后30天内死因构成

6. 术后生存状况

中国双肺脏移植受体术后30天、3个月、6个月、1年及3年生存率分别为82.1%、70.4%、63.8%、58.5%和48.4%，单肺脏移植受体相应生存率分别为85.9%、78.2%、71.4%、63.6%和44.2%，单肺脏移植受体近期生存率优于双肺脏移植受体。儿童肺脏移植术后30天、3个月、6个月及1年生存率分别为93.7%、82.0%、80.4%和80.4%。不同原发病受体的术后生存率详见表7-2。

表 7-2　中国不同特征的肺脏移植受体术后生存率

特征	30 天生存率（%）	3 个月生存率（%）	6 个月生存率（%）	1 年生存率（%）	3 年生存率（%）
移植类型					
双肺	82.1	70.4	63.8	58.5	48.4
单肺	85.9	78.2	71.4	63.6	44.2
受体年龄（岁）					
< 18	93.7	82.0	80.4	80.4	–
18 ~ 34	87.3	78.6	76.3	73.7	65.4
35 ~ 49	84.6	77.0	72.2	66.3	59.2
50 ~ 59	84.0	76.9	70.4	63.3	48.9
60 ~ 64	83.6	71.2	64.1	57.3	41.9
≥ 65	81.8	69.1	60.5	52.7	33.6
原发病					
闭塞性细支气管炎	92.4	78.3	76.7	73.3	63.5
肺尘埃沉着病	89.3	83.7	79.6	73.5	64.6
继发性肺间质纤维化	78.2	65.7	58.9	53.2	37.3
慢性阻塞性肺疾病	86.9	75.2	67.9	61.2	44.1
特发性肺间质纤维化	84.2	74.2	66.6	60.1	43.0
支气管扩张症	82.1	73.4	68.7	60.4	53.4
肺动脉高压	74.1	65.5	60.3	54.2	–
其他	76.0	65.7	58.6	53.4	45.1

四、特点与展望

1. 肺脏移植资源及移植例数稳步增长，但地区间发展差异较大

自国家卫生健康委员会启动实体器官移植资质申请认证以来，全国申报肺脏移植资质的医院数量逐年增加，通过评审获得肺脏移植资质的医院数量大幅度提升，已基本形成覆盖全国大部分地区的肺脏移植资源分布网络。但从各省具有移植资质的医疗机构数量来看，肺脏移植医疗资源分布不均衡的问题仍然存在。广州、北京、上海等一线大城市，以及沿海地区拥有的肺脏移植资源较充分，而西南地区的资源相对匮乏。

2015—2023年，全国肺脏移植开展总例数、实际开展手术的医院数量、手术量 > 10 例的医院数量及手术量 > 50 例的医院数量均呈总体上升趋势。但目前我国肺脏移植地区发展不均衡的问题仍然突出。2023 年全国实施的 959 例肺脏移植手术中，例数排名前六位医疗机构实施手术例数占到了总例数的 69.5%，手术量 > 10 例的医疗机构仅有 16 所。应采取措施进一步促进其同质化发展。

2. 肺脏移植质控体系不断完善，移植质量需不断提升

近年来，国家肺脏移植质控中心不断完善肺脏移植临床诊疗体系，推广规范化肺脏移植技术，加大宣传肺脏移植手术，推动肺脏移植数量和质量的稳步增长。纵向监测历年的移植受体术后并发症，发现移植后气道吻合口并发症发生率、移植后急性排异反应发生率均有所下降，但原发性移植物失功发生率、围手术期感染发生率有所上升。这表明需进一步加强质控指标的监测和动态反馈，持续推进全程化、多环节的术后并发症预防、控制工作机制。

我国肺脏移植与国外发达国家存在较多差别，这体现在供体、受体和术后管理多个方面。就供体而言，我国器官捐献事业还处于发展阶段，供肺情况复杂，如存在较长的机械通气时间或存在一定程度的误吸及感染，需要慎重判断其是否能够安全用于肺脏移植。就受体而言，国内诸多肺病患者年龄较大，就诊肺脏移植时病情危重，甚至达濒死状态，加之国内人口众多，会遇到各种罕见的复杂疾病，需要根据不同病情选择合适的手术时机和手术方式。在术后管理层面，我国肺脏移植术后排异反应、感染等发生率显著高于其他实体器官移植，照搬国外经验并不合适，亟须总结相关经验并制订一套适于国人的术后并发症诊治方案。我国肺脏移植手术所面临的实际困难导致了我国肺脏移植受体存活率与国际先进水平还存在一定差距，因此，构建并推广适合我国国情的肺脏移植质量控制体系是突破困境的有效途径。

3. 儿童肺脏移植快速发展，亟须总结相关经验，制订中国儿童肺脏移植行业技术文件

近年来，随着肺脏移植技术的进步和经验的积累，我国多个肺脏移植中心开展了儿童肺脏移植，尽管每年实施的儿童肺脏移植数量明显低于成人移植手术，但从2019年到2023年，中国每年开展儿童肺脏移植的数量增长了36.1%，大于成人肺脏移植的增长速度（23.8%），表明过去5年儿童肺脏移植在中国发展迅速。儿童肺脏移植总体呈现出较好的预后，术后30天存活率＞90%，提示儿童肺脏移植技术正在逐渐完善，走向成熟。儿童的免疫系统以及重要器官功能尚未完全发育成熟，肺部生长潜力与成人存在显著差异，其肺脏移植的风险和复杂性均超过成人，在手术和药物治疗过程中更容易产生并发症和不良反应，因此，亟须制订适合我国国情的儿童肺脏移植行业技术性指导文件，以促进该项技术的长足发展，提升儿童肺脏移植的长期预后。此外，中国儿童肺脏移植目前主要集中在无锡市人民医院和浙江大学医学院附属第二医院两个肺脏移植中心，提示该技术还存在较大的地区差异，有待进一步全面推广。

第八章 中国器官移植技术进展与创新

一、劈离式肝移植关键技术体系建立和推广

劈离式肝移植是外科技术层面缓解供肝短缺、扩大供肝来源的有效手段。尽管我国的肝移植已经历经40余年的发展,但既往由于供肝来源方面的限制,劈离式肝移植在国内的发展缓慢。在2015年后全面施行遗体器官捐献工作的早期,2016年劈离式肝移植占我国肝移植的比例只有1.25%,劈离式肝移植的关键技术体系亟待完善和规范。

为适应我国器官移植工作的全新发展局面,积极推动我国肝移植技术的发展创新,中山大学附属第三医院肝移植中心自2014年7月开展了首例遗体器官捐献供肝的劈离式肝移植,并持续在此领域进行了近10年的实践与探索。目前已完成了200余例的劈离式肝移植,协助和指导国内多家单位开展劈离式肝移植。开展了国内首例低龄儿童供肝(6岁4个月)完全左右半肝劈离式肝移植,全球最高龄(82岁)受体劈离式肝移植等,逐渐建立了可推广的劈离式肝移植关键技术体系(图8-1至图8-4)。

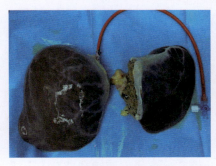

图8-1 经典离体劈离式肝移植

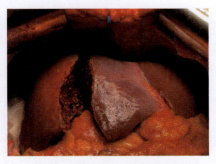

图8-2 在体完全左、右半肝劈离式肝移植

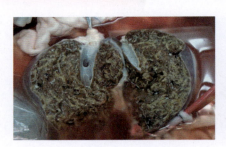
图8-3 肝中静脉正中劈分的完全左、右半肝劈离式肝移植

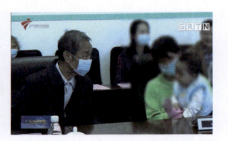
图8-4 2021年10月，完成全球最高龄受体（82岁）的劈离式肝移植，术后已经健康存活近3年

首先完善了劈离供肝的评估体系，提出了包括供体年龄、供肝脂肪变比例、供肝血管评估、供体血清钠水平和供肝超声造影评估等指标在内的可劈离供肝评估标准；完善了供肝分割、匹配、与重建方案的手术技术体系，包括经典和左右半肝劈离时血管、胆管的分割原则与血管、胆管的重建规范；同时在劈离式肝移植的供受体匹配策略、围手术期管理、并发症防治和长期随访管理等多个方面提出了相应的技术方案；并进一步对劈离供肝保存损伤控制和移植后肝脏再生的规律进行系统研究。

基于这些劈离式肝移植的理论和实践积累，积极开展相关临床和基础研究。已发表相关论文60余篇，其中在 *Hepatology*、*Journal of Hepatology*、*American Journal of Transplantation* 等领域权威杂志发表 SCI 论文30余篇。在全国同道的支持参与下，2020年牵头制定了国内首部《劈离式肝移植专家共识》，其后又牵头制定了《劈离式肝移植的供体和供肝评估专家共识》和《劈离式肝移植血管分割与重建中国专家共识》，2023年出版了国内首部《劈离式肝移植》专著。

为进一步推动劈离式肝移植的合作与发展，2020年牵头成立了我国首个劈离式肝移植技术联盟－华南劈离式肝移植联盟，并连续举办了四届全国劈离式肝移植学术论坛和三届劈离式肝移植全国学习班，有力促进了该技术在我国的应用和发展。经过同道的共同努力，2022年我国劈离式肝移植占比已经＞8%，劈离供肝占儿童肝移植的比例由2017年的8%上升至18.8%。劈离式肝移植已经成为我国肝移植的重要组成部分，也成为我国肝移植自主创新发展的重要体现。

二、甲胎蛋白－谷氨酰转肽酶－杭州标准评分（AFP-GGT-Hangzhou scoring system，AGH评分）是肝细胞癌患者肝移植术后无病生存和靶向治疗效果的预测指标

技术简介：肝移植是肝细胞癌（hepatocellular carcinoma，HCC）合并肝硬化患者最有效的根治性疗法，但移植后部分患者会出现肿瘤复发转移而严重制约疗效。然而，目前尚缺乏有效的方法来识别肝移植后HCC复发转移高风险人群，并指导辅助靶向治疗用药决策。本项目旨在通过Cox回归模型筛选复发转移相关参数，建立一个新的评分系统，用于鉴定中国人群中HCC患者肝移植术后HCC复发转移高危人群，并分析不同风险人群是否可从术后预防性使用靶向药物中获益，为辅助靶向治疗提供决策理论依据。

技术路线：回顾性收集2015年3月至2019年6月于复旦大学附属华山医院行肝移植的HCC患者的临床资料进行分析。纳入标准：①≥18岁；②病理证实HCC，且无肝外转移；③非二次移植，或肝肾联合移植；④完整的随访资料。排除标准：①术后1月内死亡；②非乙肝背景；③随访资料不全。结果：共纳入201例患者，单因素分析提示谷氨酰转移酶（GGT）＞96 U/L、甲胎蛋白（AFP）＞200 μg/L、最大肿瘤直径超过5cm、累计肿瘤直径超过8 cm、门静脉瘤栓、AJCC第八版TNM分期（Ⅲ－Ⅳ期）、超米兰标准、超UCSF标准、超杭州标准为无瘤生存的不良危险因素。多因素Cox分析提示术前甲胎蛋白（AFP）＞200 μg/L、谷氨酰转移酶（GGT）＞96 U/L、超过杭州标准是肝癌肝移植患者无瘤生存（DFS）不良的独立危险因素。基于这些因素，我们建立了AFP-GGT-杭州（AGH）评分系统，将患者分为高、中、低危组（表8-1），三组患者的总体生存（OS）率和无病生存（DFS）率差异有统计学意义（图8-5），AGH评分系统预测DFS的效能优于杭州标准、

UCSF 标准、米兰标准和 TNM 分期（图 8-6）。在高、中、低三个亚群根据使用靶向药物与否分析生存和无瘤生存的差别，仅在高危组中，我们发现仑伐替尼与对照组相比显著改善了预后（图 8-7）。

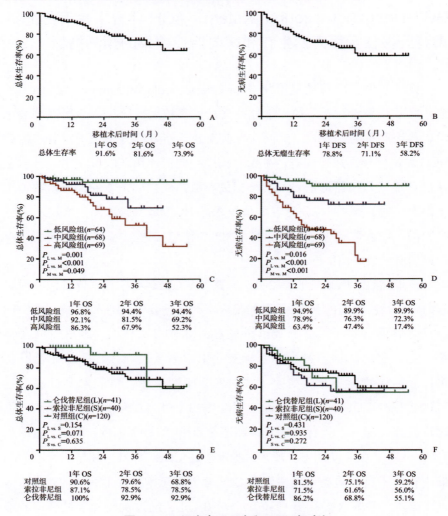

图 8-5　三组患者 OS 率和 DFS 率对比

A：整体队列的总体生存曲线；B：整体队列的总体无瘤生存曲线；C：AGH 评分高、中、低风险亚组的总体生存曲线差异；D：AGH 评分高、中、低风险亚组的总体无瘤生存曲线差异；E：总体人群中术后预防使用仑伐替尼、索拉非尼、不使用任何药物三组人群的总体生存曲线对比；F：总体人群中术后预防使用仑伐替尼、索拉非尼、不使用任何药物三组人群的总体无瘤生存曲线对比。

表 8-1　AGH 评分的定义、分级

参数	得分
AFP	
≤ 200 μg/L	1
> 200 μg/L	2
GGT	
≤ 96 U/L	1
> 96 U/L	2
是否符合杭州标准	
是	1
否	2
风险定义	
低风险	3
中风险	4
高风险	5

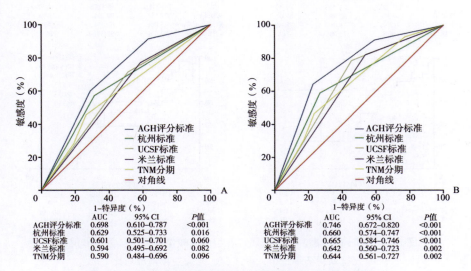

图 8-6　AGH 评分与杭州标准、米兰标准、UCSF 标准、TNM 分期的 ROC 曲线下面积比较

A：AGH 评分与杭州标准、米兰标准、UCSF 标准、TNM 分期预测总体生存的 ROC 曲线下面积比较；B：AGH 评分与杭州标准、米兰标准、UCSF 标准、TNM 分期预测无瘤生存的 ROC 曲线下面积比较。

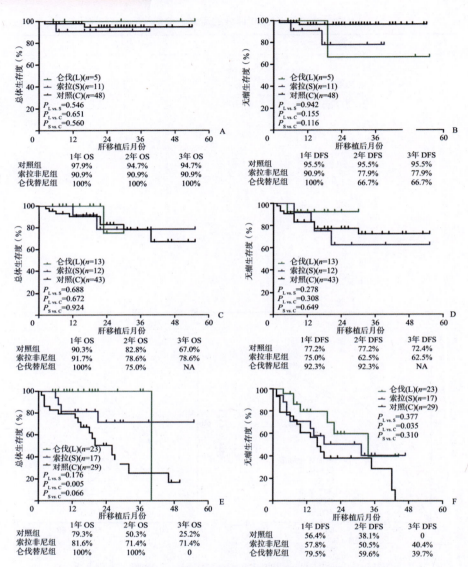

图 8-7　AGH 评分高、中、低风险亚组中比较仑伐替尼、索拉非尼、无辅助用药等三个人群生存、无瘤生存情况对比

A、B：AGH 评分低风险亚组中仑伐替尼、索拉非尼、无辅助用药等三个人群生存、无瘤生存未见显著差异；C、D：AGH 评分中风险亚组中比较仑伐替尼、索拉非尼、无辅助用药等三个人群生存、无瘤生存未见显著差异；E、F：AGH 评分高风险亚组中比较仑伐替尼、索拉非尼、无辅助用药等三个人群生存情况、无瘤生存情况对比，仑伐替尼显示出显著的生存、无瘤生存获益。

预期前景：AGH评分系统是基于中国人群开发的预测肝癌肝移植复发转移风险分层的简便、高效评分工具，并首次同时引入了针对术后靶向药物预防复发转移疗效的评价，在多中心验证后，将具有广阔的应用推广前景。

三、融合双分子标志物的肝癌肝移植患者分类新标准

肝移植是不可切除肝癌最有效的治疗手段。扩大移植受益人群、降低肿瘤复发转移、提升长期生存率一直是该领域备受关注的世界性难题。科学合理的受体筛选标准可显著提升移植疗效，实现受体最大获益。来自浙江大学的徐骁教授团队在国际上首次将双肝癌分子标志物维生素K缺乏或拮抗剂II诱导的蛋白（PIVKA-II），又称异常凝血酶原（DCP），以及甲胎蛋白（AFP）同时引入移植标准，创建全新肝癌肝移植患者分类标准和预后分层策略。

研究团队联合清华大学附属北京清华长庚医院、四川大学华西医院等国内6大肝移植中心，共纳入2015—2020年共522例肝癌肝移植病例。将肿瘤关键分子特征AFP和PIVKA-II，融合于传统肝癌结构形态学和组织病理学等重要特征，提出肝癌肝移植患者分类新标准（HC&PIVKA-II）。与传统移植标准相比，HC&PIVKA-II进一步扩大了21.6%的肝移植受益人群，且1、3、5年总体生存率不存在显著差异，分别为89.4%、79.9%和78.7%（图8-8）。

研究成果在国际外科学期刊 *International Journal of Surgery* 上发表。该成果紧密围绕当前肝癌肝移植临床瓶颈难题，基于中国多中心肝移植列队，进一步突破了传统移植标准的局限性，丰富了肝癌肝移植个体化精准治疗新体系的内涵，在国际"移植肿瘤学"领域贡献了中国经验。

杭州标准和PIVKA-II：（A）累计肿瘤直径≤8 cm；（B）累计肿瘤直径>8 cm，肿瘤组织学分化等级为中高分化，且满足以下任一条件：

（B1）PIVKA-II浓度≤240 mAU/mL；（B2）AFP浓度≤400 ng/mL。

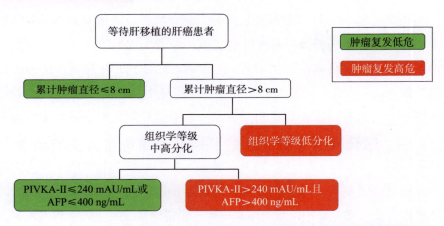

图 8-8 融合 PIVKA-II 和 AFP 双分子标志物的肝癌肝移植患者分类新标准

四、天然高分子生物肝材料治疗多器官功能衰竭核心技术体系的建立与应用

肝功能衰竭是严重危害人类健康的重大疾病。我国是世界上肝功能衰竭最严重的国家之一，每年各种原因导致的急慢性肝功能衰竭新发病人数 > 300 万，传统内科治疗效果有限，难以阻止疾病恶化，患者死亡率高达 50% ~ 90%，重症肝功能衰竭患者 3 个月死亡率高达 80%。降低肝功能衰竭病死率是健康中国战略的重大需求。肝功能失代偿产生的毒性代谢产物是多器官功能衰竭的常见始动因素。人工肝可有效清除机体毒素，为肝脏再生、脏器功能恢复创造有利条件，是肝功能衰竭患者的替代疗法，更是器官移植的桥梁。但现有人工肝产品的安全性和有效性难以兼具，且多以国外产品为主，关键技术壁垒高，费用高昂，是我国"卡脖子"技术之一。因此，开发安全高效人工肝产品仍是目前研发的重点，是该行业发展的突破口。

本项目组针对重症肝功能衰竭患者（MELD ≥ 30）移植等待期间死亡率高及移植术后效果差等"瓶颈"问题，历经 10 余年跨学科交叉合作研究，创建了天然高分子生物肝材料治疗多器官功能衰竭核心技术体系，创新研发了甲壳素等新型天然高分子血液净化吸附材料，可安全、高效、精准吸附胆红素/血氨/肌酐/尿酸/内毒素等多器官功能衰竭代谢毒素，解决了人工肝吸附材料高效性和安全性难以兼具的关键技术问题，可用于改善患者内环境，优化供体与器官质量，助力于多器官功能衰竭疾病治疗的攻坚克难。研发了新型生物人工肝反应器并创建甲壳素基细胞微载体、改良型肝细胞及机械灌注的"三位一体"天然高分子生物人工肝系统，显著增加肝细胞在反应器内的可贴壁面积，加大细胞装载量，提高物质的交换效率，改善细胞培养环境，提高肝细胞活性，解决了传统生物人工肝肝细胞黏附和活力差的问题，大幅度提高了胆红素等毒素的清除率。临床试验结果显示，天然高分子生物人工肝系统明显改善患者的内环境和肝功能，可将 MELD ≥ 30 分患者死亡率由 77% 降至 50%，将该类患者肝移植术后 1 年存活率提高至 91%（国际报道 58%~65%），降低治疗费用近 50%，造福广大患者（图 8-9）。

　　研究成果经第三方科技评价，整体达到国际领先水平。该项目获授权专利 24 项（发明专利 17 项，实用新型 7 项），部分已完成临床转化，获批湖北省卫生健康委员会新增医疗服务定价收费项目，并已在国家医保局备案；研究平台获批湖北省天然高分子生物肝临床医学研究中心；系列成果获批国家自然科学基金、湖北省科技创新专项、湖北省自然科学基金等 20 余项相关科研项目支持；代表性成果发表于 *Advanced Materials*、*Advanced Functional Material*、*SusMat*、*Carbohydrate Polymers*、*Journal of Materials Chemistry B* 等期刊。作为国家人体捐献器官获取质量控制中心、湖北省天然高分子生物肝临床医学研究中心、湖北省肝胆疾病学会主委单位，成果在全国 20 余家大型三甲医院推广应用。研究成果获得 CCTV-10 科教频道《走进科学》栏目三期专题报道；临床治疗效果被人民网等多家权威媒体报道。成果荣获第九届"创青春"中国青年创新创业大赛全国金奖和 2022 年度湖北省科学技术发明奖一等奖。

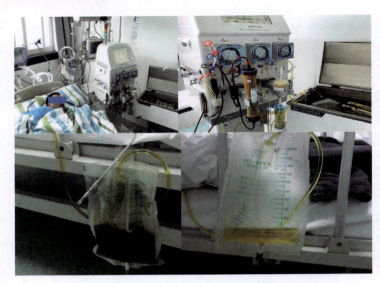

图 8-9 天然高分子生物人工肝系统及其临床治疗效果

五、基于基因模型指导肝移植术后抗排异反应精准给药方案

技术简介：肝移植的成功取决于在充分的免疫抑制与免疫抑制药物相关的毒副作用最小化之间实现良好的平衡，但患者之间的免疫抑制剂剂量差异高达 20 倍（0.5 ~ 10 mg/d），很难确定免疫抑制剂的最佳初始剂量。供肝和受体两套基因组的相互作用是造成个体间免疫抑制剂代谢差异的主要原因，对其代谢变异解释度 > 50%。通过药物基因组学、药物代谢动力学及生物信息学分析构建了包括主效基因（供、受体 CYP3A5 rs776746）、微效基因（受体 SLCO1B1 rs4149015、受体 CHST10 rs4149015）、受体总胆红素及体重在内的他克莫司首剂用药模型，借助自主研发的全自动用药智能一体机能够准确区分受体的代谢类型，并通过创建的肝移植术后个体化用药网站，提供精确的个体化初始给药剂量，为临床肝移植患者个性化精准给药提供依据。经多中心、单盲、随机对照临床试验（ChiCTR2100050288）验证结果显示基于模型指导用药患者

间他克莫司首剂剂量差异高达 4.2 倍（0.023～0.096 mg/kg），模型指导用药能够显著减少调药次数（2.75±2.01 vs. 6.05±3.35），提高肝移植术后 24 h 内血药浓度达标率（75% vs. 40%，P=0.025），并能够降低肝移植术后急性排异反应的发生率和药物的毒性及不良反应（图 8-10）。

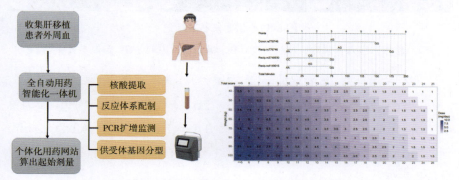

图 8-10　技术路线

阶段性进展及预期前景：相关研究结果发表在柳叶刀子刊 *eClinicalMedicine* 杂志，据此研发精准用药智能化一体机，并已获得国家发明专利（专利号：ZL 2021 1 1211804.2），目前已在多家肝移植中心推广应用。

六、达芬奇机器人辅助腹腔镜技术在肾移植中的应用

技术简介：为减少肾移植手术创伤及切口并发症，昆明市第一人民医院结合传统开放手术及达芬奇机器人在外科手术中的特殊优势，于 2019 年 2 月 3 日开展了我国首例机器人 DD 肾移植术。经过不断优化及持续改进机器人肾移植手术流程，形成了一套标准的机器人辅助腹腔镜肾移植手术体系。目前为国内开展机器人 DD 肾移植手术例数最多的中心，并于 2023 年 4 月由清华大学出版社出版《机器人肾移植手术学》一书。

技术路线：

（1）供肾修整后放入自制肾袋，标记移植肾及血管方向（图 8-11A、图 8-11B），自制单孔平台（图 8-11C）。

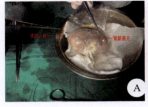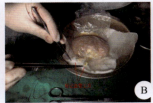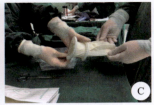

图 8-11　供肾修整及标记

A：移植肾装入肾袋内，标记方向；B：标记血管方向；C：自制单孔平台。

（2）全麻插管，患者取仰卧位，两腿分开，头低脚高 30°（图 8-12A）。

（3）腹部置入 6 个 Trocar（图 8-12B），气腹压 13 mmHg，C 为镜头 Trocar，R1、R2、R3 分别为机械臂 8 mm Trocar，A1、A2 为 12 mm 辅助 Trocar。取下腹正中 5～7 cm 切口，置入自制单孔平台（图 8-12C），对接机械臂（图 8-13A）。

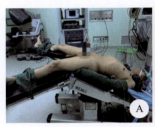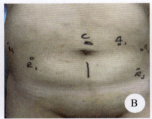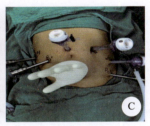

图 8-12　腹部 Trocar 位置

A：机器人肾移植体位；B：Trocar 位置；C：置入 Trocar 及自制通道。

（4）沿侧腹壁切开腹膜，上至回盲部上方约 3 cm，下至脐正中韧带下方（图 8-13B），建立肾巢。在腹膜外游离髂外动、静脉。通过单孔平台放入常温纱布垫（图 8-13C）、将移植肾置入纱布垫上，确认移植肾方向，避免上下极颠倒。先阻断髂外静脉，根据移植肾静脉直径纵行剪开受体髂外静脉，肝素盐水反复冲洗静脉管腔，采用 Gore-Tex CV-6 血管缝线端侧吻合移植肾静脉与髂外静脉（图 8-13D）。在静脉吻合完成之前，注入肝素盐水再次冲洗静脉管腔，阻断移植肾静脉，打开髂外静脉的血管阻断夹，试漏。同样方法行移植肾动脉和受体的髂外动脉端侧吻合（图 8-13E）。术中通过单孔平台向自制肾袋内加冰屑，保证移植肾开放

第八章 中国器官移植技术进展与创新

之前持续低温。依次开放移植肾静脉、移植肾动脉（图 8-13F），观察移植肾再灌注及输尿管排尿情况，将移植肾移入肾巢内。纵行切开膀胱后底壁（移植肾摆放侧）约 2.0 cm，4-0 可吸收线进行移植肾输尿管、膀胱再植（图 8-13G），输尿管内留置 5F 输尿管支架。关闭侧腹膜（图 8-13H），将移植肾、移植输尿管完全腹膜外化（图 8-13I）。

阶段性进展或该项目的预期前景等：目前昆明市第一人民医院共完成机器人肾移植术 121 例，其中机器人 DD 肾移植 98 例，机器人亲体肾移植 23 例，均顺利完成，无中转开放病例。开放肾移植手术组和机器人肾移植手术组总手术时间、动脉吻合时间、静脉吻合时间、输尿管吻合时间、失血量、肌酐恢复情况比较，差异均无统计的意义（$P > 0.05$）；机器人肾移植手术组住院时间、术后切口疼痛情况优于开放手术组。初步结论：机器人辅助腹腔镜下肾移植术安全、可靠，可达到与开放手术相同的肾功能恢复效果，同时加快患者术后恢复。

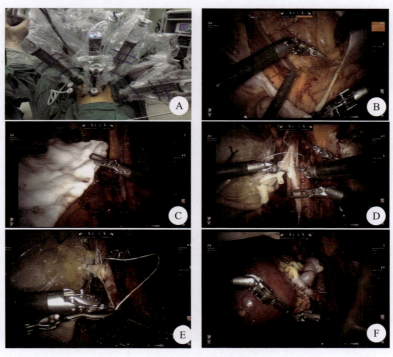

图 8-13　手术过程

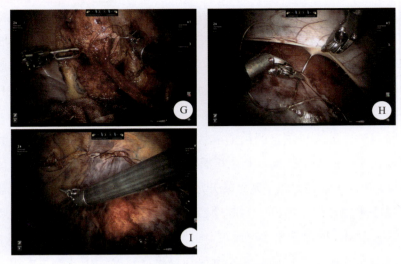

图 8-13 （续）

A：对接机械臂；B：沿侧腹壁切开腹膜；C：置入纱布垫；D：吻合移植肾静脉与髂外静脉；E：吻合移植动脉与髂外动脉；F：移植肾血管开放；G：膀胱输尿管吻合；H：缝合腹膜；I：移植肾腹膜外化。

七、人工血管保护外鞘预防移植肾动脉扭折的疗效

移植肾动脉扭折是肾移植较为少见而严重的并发症，如果术中、术后发现此类情况，常需要再次手术重新吻合。在术中发现移植肾动脉扭折后采用人工血管包裹移植肾动脉可有效改善移植肾动脉扭折状态，避免二次手术。

2019年1月至2022年6月苏州大学附属第一医院泌尿外科共8例肾移植术中发现移植肾动脉扭折，采用人工血管包裹移植肾动脉，纠正动脉走行，并纳入研究。所有患者均采用右下腹斜切口暴露髂血管，动脉与静脉分别采用髂内动脉端端吻合和髂外静脉端侧吻合。移植肾放于右髂窝后，观察动脉出现明显扭折（图8-14A）。遂采用长约5 cm、直径8 mm人工血管（根据动脉长度直径决定型号），纵向剪开（图8-14B）包裹于动脉，间断缝合人工血管纵行切口后再次将移植肾摆放于右髂窝

（图8-14C），观察血管走行及移植肾血供状态。

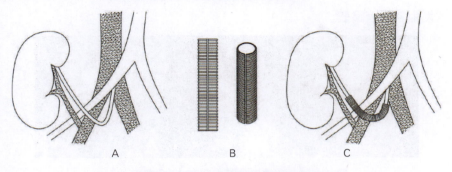

图8-14 人工血管外鞘手术示意图

7例患者术后尿量、肾功能正常恢复；1例发生DGF 2周时肾功能恢复正常。围手术期均无急性排异、发热、切口或肺部感染等并发症发生。术后第1天、7天、14天行移植肾彩超或造影评估血流，未见明显异常。

所有患者随访至今，无移植肾区不适。定期复查移植肾彩超，未见移植肾动脉狭窄。复查盆腔CT，人工血管鞘在位良好，无渗出移位（图8-15）。

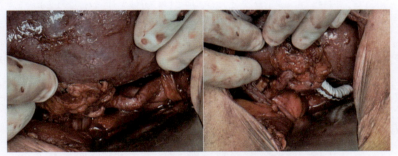

图8-15 术中移植肾动脉扭结及人工血管外鞘放置

ePTFE人工血管由合成无纺材料聚四氟乙烯制成，产品上标有蓝色指示线，以及聚四氟乙烯支撑环（图8-16），具柔韧性、富有弹性、可任意弯曲而不瘪塌且具有一定的顺应性及较强的生物相容性，目前多广泛用于临床血管替代治疗，而作为移植肾动脉外鞘使用，目前国内外鲜有报道。该外鞘对移植肾动脉起到了良好的支撑作用，从而使扭折的动脉呈自然弧形，本研究中8例患者动脉包裹后均获得了良好的走行。

ePTFE 人工血管较强的生物相容性及本身具备的抗感染能力，使其感染的发生率极大降低。

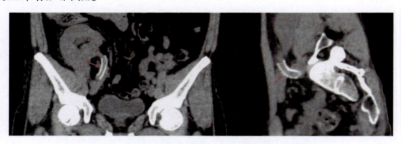

图 8-16　人工血管外鞘（ＣＴ轴位及矢状位）

综上所述，肾移植术中若遇到移植肾动脉扭折时，ePTFE 人工血管作为外鞘可有效纠正移植肾动脉走行，减少移植肾动脉狭窄可能。该方法操作简单、安全性高、并发症少。不足之处在于人工血管价格昂贵。

八、六基因编辑猪 - 恒河猴异种肾脏移植

空军军医大学第一附属医院泌尿外科于 2023 年 10 月 27 日进行了多基因编辑猪 – 恒河猴的异种肾脏移植实验。研究以 6 基因编辑猪作为供体，供体猪使用 CRISPR/Cas9 技术敲除了可能引起超急性排异反应的糖类抗原，并通过转基因技术表达 2 种人补体调节蛋白及 1 种人凝血调节蛋白。研究团队将供体猪的左肾移植至受体猴的右侧腹腔，移植肾动、静脉分别以端 – 侧吻合法缝合至受体的腹主动脉及下腔静脉，移植肾在血流开放后立刻有尿液产生。移植肾输尿管采用 Lich–Gregoir 法吻合至受体膀胱。手术同期切除了受体猴的自体双肾，使异种移植肾完全承担调节水、电解质平衡的功能，充分模拟临床中尿毒症患者的情形。围术期使用了抗胸腺细胞免疫球蛋白、抗 CD20 单抗、补体清除在内的免疫抑制诱导方案，而免疫抑制维持方案则使用与临床相同的"他克莫司 + 吗替麦考酚酯 + 糖皮质激素"的三联免疫抑制方案（图 8-17）。

移植肾在术后第 1 周内功能良好，每日尿量波动于 585～2 543 mL，血肌酐维持在正常水平，其间，多普勒彩超显示移植肾血流灌注良好

（图8-18）。术后第9天起受体猴出现尿量减少、血肌酐升高，穿刺提示"急性抗体介导的排异反应"。经糖皮质激素冲击、抗CD20单抗、静注免疫球蛋白等治疗后无明显好转，再次进行移植肾穿刺活检提示"急性抗体介导排异反应较前加重"。最终考虑逆转排异困难，于术后27天对受体猴实施安乐死。

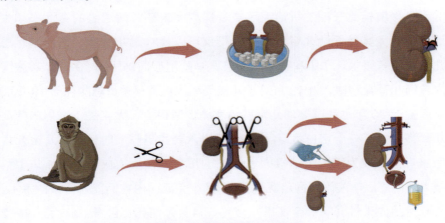

图8-17 实验设计示意图

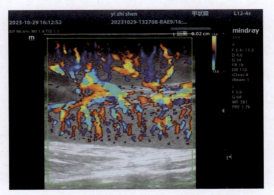

图8-18 术后彩色多普勒显示移植肾血流灌注良好

本研究证实了使用多基因编辑猪作为供体，并使用临床常规使用的免疫抑制诱导和维持方案预防了超急性排异反应的发生，并实现了受体猴较长时间的存活，达到国内异种肾移植报道中较领先水平。但本研究仍未避免抗体介导的排异反应的发生，这可能与免疫抑制方案中缺乏阻断共刺激通路的药物有关。在未来的研究中，将进一步优化研究方案，以延长多基因编辑猪-恒河猴异种肾脏移植的存活时间，并为异种移植最终进入临床提供经验。

九、国内首组婴幼儿供肾给婴幼儿肾移植 37 例

肾移植相比长期透析治疗可显著提高终末期肾病患者的存活率和生活质量，尤其是低龄儿童肾移植，不仅可以挽救患儿生命，亦能满足患儿生长发育需求。华中科技大学同济医学院附属同济医院 1979 年实施国内首例儿童肾移植，为 19 月龄患儿接受成人供肾移植，患儿存活 10 年。之后的近 30 年，我国婴幼儿肾移植实施例数极少，尤其是 1 岁以内的婴儿肾移植一直处于空白状态。2015 年进入器官捐献新时代后，儿童死亡后器官捐献成为可能，这极大地促进了儿童肾移植的快速发展。华中科技大学同济医学院附属同济医院于 2017 年完成国内首例婴儿肾移植手术，为 6 月龄先天性肾病综合征患儿接受 5 月龄外伤死亡供肾，此后至 2022 年 7 月 31 日期间，已累计实施 < 3 岁的儿童肾移植 37 例（占国内绝大多数），其中 < 1 岁的婴儿肾移植 13 例（35.1%），< 6 月龄小婴儿肾移植 7 例（18.9%），年龄最小受体仅 2 个月 26 天、体重 3.2 kg，为成功开展的世界最小年龄儿童肾移植案例。

37 例婴幼儿受体中位年龄 16 个月（范围：2 个月 26 天至 36 个月），中位体重 8 kg（范围：3.2～14.0 kg）。供肾全部来自儿童死亡后器官捐献，除 1 个供体年龄为 10 岁外，其余所有供体的年龄 ≤ 3 岁，最小年龄 9 天，中位年龄 7 个月（图 8-19A），最小体重 2.8 kg，中位体重 6.0 kg（图 8-19B）。受体原发病最多见为先天性肾病综合征（13 例，41.9%）。19 例次（51.3%）为腹腔内移植，余 18 例次（48.6%）为髂窝内移植。移植肾 1 年、2 年存活率均为 85.3%，移植受体 1 年、2 年存活率均为 96.8%（图 8-20）。

虽然婴幼儿肾移植手术及术后管理难度极大，本研究仍取得了与国际水平相比更优的移植效果。说明利用婴幼儿供肾，经过精细的手术及术后多学科协作管理，婴幼儿肾移植能够取得相对满意的临床效果。本

组病例实践为我国乃至全球的低龄患儿利用婴幼儿供肾实施移植提供了宝贵的早期经验。

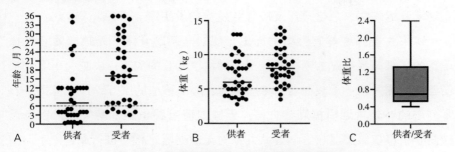

图 8-19　肾移植供体及受体年龄及体重分布

A：供体和受体年龄分布；B：供体和受体体重分布；C：供/受体体重比；A 及 B 中显示供体为 36 例，1 例 10 岁供体未在图中显示。

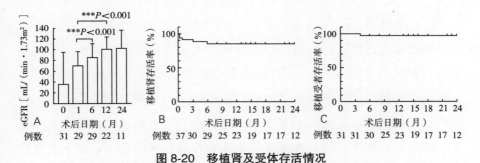

图 8-20　移植肾及受体存活情况

A：肾移植后估算肾小球滤过率（eGFR）变化情况；B：移植物存活生存曲线；C：受体存活生存曲线。

十、无缺血心脏移植

2021 年 6 月 26 日，中山大学附属第一医院成功完成全球首例无缺血心脏移植手术，患者实现长期生存。殷胜利教授作为主要作者之一，于 2022 年在 *The Lancet Regional Health-Western Pacific* 发表论文 *Transplantation of a Beating Heart: A first in Man*，并于 2023 年参与撰写并出版《无缺血器官移植》一书。无缺血器官移植通过体外常温机械灌注支持及创新性手术方式，实现供体器官获取与受体器官植入全程血流不中断、器官始终保有血液与氧气供应，从根本上消除了器官获取与移植过程中缺血-再灌注损伤对器官功能的影响，显著降低了器官移植术后器官功能延迟恢复、急性排斥反应等并发症的发生率。

本书主要围绕器官移植的历史、现状与问题介绍；无缺血器官移植理念的详细阐释；缺血-再灌注损伤对移植器官的危害；缺血-再灌注损伤与免疫的关系；无缺血器官（肝、肾、心）移植的展开论述，包括肝、肾、心的体外常温机械灌注方法；无缺血器官移植的麻醉管理；以及无缺血器官移植展望器官医学等共九章对无缺血器官移植进行阐述。

十一、一种全新的心肌活检技术在心脏移植术后的应用

1. 技术简介

心脏移植是治疗各种终末期心脏病的有效方法，而排异反应仍是患者死亡的主要原因之一。心肌活检是诊断排异反应的"金"标准。目前临床上常用的心内膜心肌活检是在放射线下，利用导管式活检钳，经周围血管到达右心室或左心室夹取心内膜心肌组织的技术，因技术难度高，单次活检病理组织标本量少，能独立开展的医院较少，该技术开展受限。

2023年，武汉亚洲心脏病医院采用了一种全新的心肌活检方法，即超声引导下经皮穿刺室间隔内心肌活检术，现将这一技术的操作以及优缺点进行总结。

2. 技术路线

1）操作过程（技术路线见图8-21、图8-22）

（1）按照全麻准备，术前禁食12h，禁饮4~6h；签署知情同意书。

（2）患者取左侧卧位，右肩部垫高30°~40°，静脉全身麻醉经喉罩通气。

（3）用Philip EPIQ7c超声机器，先将S5-1超声探头用无菌袖保护，消毒铺巾后，在超声探头上加载LEAPMED A型穿刺引导架（3 530），

第八章 中国器官移植技术进展与创新

经胸超声明确穿刺路径上无冠脉血管后，确定好进针路线，将 Bard Mission Disposable Core Biopsy Instrument 放进 LEAPMED A 型穿刺架的 17G 卡槽，沿着超声已经确定的穿刺路线进针，依次穿破皮肤、肋间肌肉、心包和心尖部室壁肌肉至室间隔内。

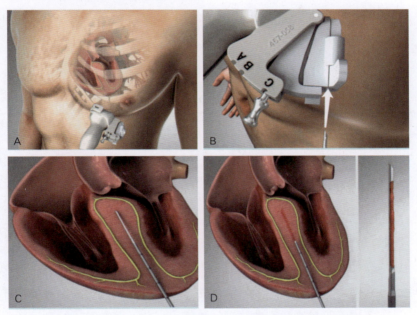

图 8-21　超声引导下经皮穿刺室间隔内心肌活检术模拟图

A：超声定位，确定穿刺路径；B：活检针插入引导架卡槽中；C：活检针进入室间隔内；D：活检针采样。

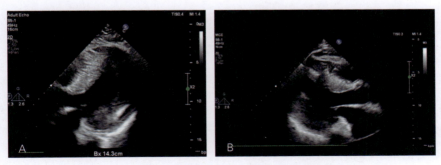

图 8-22　超声引导下经皮穿刺室间隔内心肌活检术

A：超声定位，确定穿刺路径；B：进针及采样。

（4）取走穿刺引导的卡槽，然后再次通过超声确定活检针位于室间隔内，位置距离左、右心室内膜面 > 3 mm，尖端距离主动脉瓣环 > 20 mm，启动活检针，一次性获取室间隔内心肌组织 10 mm×1 mm。

（5）退针，将心肌组织从活检针的槽孔中取出，送病理科进行病检。

（6）超声实时观察 5～10 min，确定无心包积液后，穿刺点局部消毒包扎，患者清醒后回病房。

2）优缺点比较（表 8-2）

表 8-2　优缺点比较

	优点	缺点
DSA 下经导管 EMB	局麻，历史悠久	DSA 射线，单次取样量少 右室损伤，心包积液，盲抓取，费用高
超声引导下经室间隔内 MB	超声引导，无辐射，可视化 一次取样量大，并发症少 学习曲线短，费用低	新技术，全麻和超声科合作

3. 阶段性进展及预期前景

武汉亚洲心脏病医院已经成功实施该技术 15 例，全部成功，例均手术时间 5～10 min，1 例（ECMO 辅助患者）发生心包积液，其他无并发症。该方法操作简单，学习曲线短，具有可视化、可重复、绿色无辐射、单次活检标本量大等特点，相比传统方法有显著优势，在心脏移植术后心肌活检上具有可推广性和广泛应用的空间。

十二、基于机器学习的肺移植患者预后模型

近年来，我国肺移植在手术技术和围术期管理方面已经取得了巨大进步，但肺移植受体的生存结果仍不令人满意。如何提高受体远期生存和生活质量是世界范围内肺移植领域高度关注的问题。开发准确的生存预测工具对移植医生制订个体化管理方案进而改善受体预后至关重要。在这一背景下，陈静瑜教授及其团队，基于中国肺移植临床数据，首次利用人工智能方法构建了肺移植受体术后连续生存的预后模型，利用随

机生存森林（random survival forests，RSF）这一机器学习算法，开发并验证了一种预测肺移植受体总体生存的预后模型。研究发现，RSF 模型对肺移植术后受体的生存结果具有很好的预测性能，其整合曲线下面积（iAUC）值高达 0.879。此外，在相同的建模特征下，RSF 的预测性能远优于传统 Cox 回归模型。值得注意的是，根据 RSF 模型预测的最佳阈值，可将肺移植受体进行预后分层，其中低风险组和高风险组的总体生存具有显著差异，平均总生存期分别为 52.9 个月和 14.8 个月。这一结果表明人工智能方法在肺移植领域具有巨大潜力，为后续研究提供了重要前期基础，同时也促进了该方法的临床应用。该人工智能模型可为移植医生的管理决策提供实用、可靠的指导，最终整体上改善肺移植术后受体的远期生存和生活质量。

2023 年 5 月 5 日，该研究被美国医学会（JAMA）子刊 *JAMA Network Open* IF：13.88，中国科学院分区 1 区刊载，是我国肺移植临床数据首次破冰被国际顶级期刊接受。这对于我国肺移植临床医学领域的发展具有重要意义，也为今后我国肺移植临床实践提供了宝贵的经验和指导。由于历史原因，国际上仍有部分组织或个人仍然对我国器官移植工作带有偏见。陈静瑜团队此次研究成果能被 JAMA 子刊接受，表明了我国肺移植工作已逐渐被国际认可，也证明了我国肺移植的临床研究水平逐渐靠近国际前列，极大促进了我国肺移植的对外交流和合作。

十三、机器人辅助微创入路单肺移植手术

1. 技术简介

目前，大多数肺移植手术通过开放切口（如横断胸骨 Clam shell 切口、标准后外侧切口等）实施双肺或单肺移植手术。而这些手术方式创伤大、胸壁呼吸肌损伤大、术后疼痛明显、皮肤或胸骨切口相关并发症多，影响患者的术后康复和生活质量。相比传统切口肺移植手术，机器人辅助微创入路肺移植手术的优势主要体现在以下方面：

（1）手术切口微创，助力术后加速康复。机器人辅助微创手术切口小，创伤小，呼吸肌功能保护良好，疼痛相对较轻，患者术后呼吸、咳痰有力，加速了术后康复。

（2）缝合精准，降低操作难度。肺脏移植手术最关键的就是支气管、肺动脉和左房袖的吻合。而达芬奇机器人手术系统最大的优势正在于狭小空间的复杂操作如缝合。通过三维高清视野和灵活的机械臂末端器械，主刀医生可以全方位、无死角、精准、快速地进行支气管、肺动脉和左房袖的吻合。

（3）止血彻底，提高安全性。在机器人辅助肺移植手术中，通过三维高清视野，可以更精准地剥离粘连带，清楚观察每个出血点，做到精准、确切、充分地止血。

2. 技术路线

青岛大学附属医院充分利用达芬奇机器人的三维高清视野和灵活旋转的机械手腕等优势，完成高难度解剖、可靠止血、精准吻合。在机器人辅助微创肺移植手术中，吻合操作（包括支气管、肺动脉、左心房袖）均使用半连续缝合方法。全部手术核心操作包括缝合和打结，都是由主刀操控机器人手臂完成。此外，为了应对术中突发情况，手术助手需要经过高水平的培训，能够独立进行肺部微创手术（图8-23）。

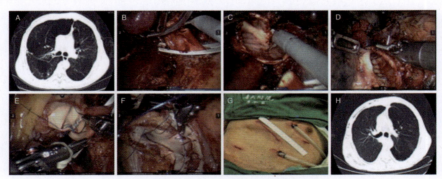

图8-23　肺部微创手术

A：受体术前胸部计算机断层扫描；B：机器人剪刀剪开肺动脉；C：机器人剪刀剪开右主支气管；D：支气管行端-端半连续吻合术；E：肺动脉吻合术；F：左心房吻合术；G：皮内缝合手术皮肤切口；H：受体术后胸部计算机断层扫描。

青岛大学附属医院胸外科矫文捷主任团队于2022年4月成功开展亚洲首例机器人辅助单肺移植手术，随访至今27个月。

2023年2月在 Chinese Medical Journal 杂志公开发表世界首篇机器人辅助单肺移植手术文章。

十四、供体来源游离 DNA 在肺移植术后排异反应诊断中的应用

供体来源游离 DNA（donor-derived cell-free DNA，dd-cfDNA）是指器官移植术后供体循环体液中来自凋亡或坏死供体细胞的游离 DNA，其带有供体的组织细胞信息。近年来 dd-cfDNA 成为实体器官移植领域的研究热点，集中成果发表让移植领域对 dd-cfDNA 在移植物损伤特别是急性排异方面的认识不断深入，dd-cfDNA 有望成为未来肺移植排异无创检测的生物标志物。然而国内肺移植领域尚无相关研究。

广州医科大学附属第一医院肺移植团队率先在中国肺移植受体中开展了两项 dd-cfDNA 相关的回顾性临床研究，第一项研究共纳入了170例肺移植受体，分为感染、急性排异反应、慢性移植肺失功（chronic lung allograft dysfunction，CLAD）及稳定组，比较四组间血浆 dd-cfDNA 水平差异，发现急排组及 CLAD 组 dd-cfDNA 显著高于感染及稳定组（图8-24A），以1.17%作为阈值，dd-cfDNA 诊断急排的敏感性和特异性分别为89.19%和86.47%。同时 dd-cfDNA 水平在治疗前后存在显著差异，治疗后 dd-cfDNA 水平明显下降（图8-24B、C）。该研究是国内首个探索 dd-cfDNA 在肺移植受体诊断中应用的研究，为 dd-cfDNA 用于无创监测肺移植受体病情奠定基础。第二项研究是在第一项研究的基础上，首次将 dd-cfDNA 的结果与肺泡灌洗液（BALF）的宏基因组二代测序（mNGS）结果进行关联分析，共纳入肺移植受体188例，分为排异、感染及稳定三组。研究发现肺移植受体中，血浆 dd-cfDNA 水平随时间推移不断下降，不发生排异反应时，大约于术后1个月达到稳定（图8-24D）；

在感染组中，巨细胞病毒感染后dd-cfDNA升高，而细菌、真菌感染则无明显变化；dd-cfDNA与mNGS结果联合可以显著提高dd-cfDNA对排异反应的诊断效能，dd-cfDNA升高而mNGS结果阴性对排异反应诊断的阳性预测值和阴性预测值分别为88.7%和99.2%（图8-24E）。

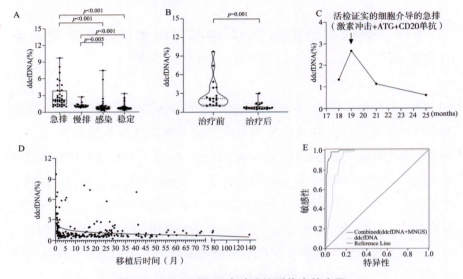

图8-24　dd-cfDNA在肺移植受体中的应用

A：不同组间血浆dd-cfDNA含量；B：血浆dd-cfDNA治疗后显著降低；C：肺组织病理证实的3级排异反应，治疗前dd-cfDNA显著升高，随治疗好转，dd-cfDNA逐渐下降；D：肺移植受体中，血浆dd-cfDNA含量随时间推移逐渐降低，大约术后1个月达到稳态；E：dd-cfDNA与mNGS结果联合可提高dd-cfDNA诊断排异反应敏感性及特异性。

综上，该研究是首个中国肺移植受体dd-cfDNA的研究，提供了中国肺移植受体dd-cfDNA的基线数据，初步阐述了dd-cfDNA在肺移植术后并发症诊断中的应用，为dd-cfDNA作为无创手段监测肺移植术后并发症的应用奠定了基础。

索 引

中文全称	英文全称	缩写	页码
国家人体捐献器官获取质量控制中心	National Quality Control Center for Donated Organ Procurement	OPQC	11
功能延迟性恢复	delayed graft function	DGF	10
原发性无功能	primary nonfunction	PNF	10
每百万人口遗体器官捐献率	Organ Donation Per Million Population	PMP	5
纽约心脏病学会	New York Heart Association	NYHA	64
脑死亡供体	donors after brain death	DBD	14
脑－心双死亡供体	donors after brain and circulatory death	DBCD	14
劈离式肝脏移植	split liver transplantation	SLT	39
亲属间活体肝脏移植	living related donor liver transplantation	LDLT	33
人体器官获取组织	Organ Procurement Organization	OPO	10
体外膜氧合	extracorporeal membrane oxygenation	ECMO	19
体重指数	body mass index	BMI	35
心脏死亡供体	donors after circulatory death	DCD	14
遗体器官捐献	deceased donation	DD	41
遗体器官捐献肝脏移植	deceased donor liver transplantation	DDLT	33
中国肝移植注册系统	China Liver Transplant Registry	CLTR	32
中国人体器官分配与共享计算机系统	China Organ Transplant Response System	COTRS	9
重症监护室	intensive care unit	ICU	64

Chapter 1   Human Organ Donation in China

Organ donation is a commendable endeavor that fosters boundless love among humanity and saves lives that are on the brink of danger. The significance of organ donation was further underscored by the *Regulations on Human Organ Donation and Transplantation* (hereinafter referred to as the *Regulations*), which was approved by the 17th Executive Meeting of the State Council of the People's Republic of China on October 20th, 2023. The Regulations mandate that organ donation should comply with the principles of gratuity and voluntariness, and the conditions and procedure for organ donation should be refined in accordance with the *Civil Code of the People's Republic of China*. In addition, it mandates that the state should enhance the popularization of knowledge, education, and publicity regarding organ donation, and that news media should conduct public campaigns on the subject for cultivating a social environment that is supportive of organ donation. Furthermore, the *Regulations* encourage organ donation from deceased individuals and strengthen commendation and guidance provided in this regard. The Central Committee of the Communist Party of China and the State Council attach great importance to the development of human organ donation and transplantation, and health departments and Red Cross Societies at all levels have worked in unity and coordination, actively explored and innovated, and have established and continuously improved the working system for human organ donation. Extensive efforts have been made in promoting the concept of organ donation, facilitating organ donation volunteer registry, witnessing donation process, organizing commemorating activities and providing humanitarian care related work. Remarkable results have been made in improving the organizational network on human organ donation, as well as establishment and management of coordinator teams.

1.1 Organizations and team building

1.1.1 Organizations

In 2023, three provincial-level Red Cross Societies in Jilin, Henan, and Gansu, established new administrative agencies for human organ donation. As of the end of 2023, a total of 30 provincial-level Red Cross Societies across the country had established such administrative agencies (Table 1-1).

Table 1-1　Establishment of provincial-level Red Cross Societies human organ donation administrative agencies nationwide by the end of 2023

No.	Provinces (Autonomous regions/ Municipalities)	Name of institutions
1	Beijing	Donation Service Center, Red Cross Society of China Beijing Branch
2	Tianjin	Tianjin Red Cross Affairs Center
3	Hebei	Hebei Red Cross Society Blood, Stem Cells and Organ Donation Center
4	Shanxi	Shanxi Red Cross Society Social Work Service Center
5	Inner Mongolia	Inner Mongolia Autonomous Region Red Cross Society Donation Service Center
6	Liaoning	Liaoning Provincial Red Cross Society Development and Service Center
7	Jilin	Jilin Provincial Red Cross Society Donation Service Center
8	Heilongjiang	Heilongjiang Red Cross Society Disaster Preparedness and Organ Donation Center
9	Shanghai	Shanghai Red Cross Affairs Center

Chapter 1 Human Organ Donation in China

Continued

No.	Provinces (Autonomous regions/Municipalities)	Name of institutions
10	Jiangsu	Jiangsu Provincial Human Organ Donation Administrative Center
11	Zhejiang	Zhejiang Provincial Human Organ Donation Administrative Center
12	Anhui	Anhui Red Cross Society Blood, Stem Cells and Organ Donation Office
13	Fujian	Fujian Provincial Human Organ Donation Administrative Center
14	Jiangxi	Jiangxi Red Cross Society Humanitarian Rescue Service Center
15	Shandong	Shandong Red Cross Society Medical Donation Service Center
16	Henan	Henan Provincial Human Organ Donation Administrative Office
17	Hubei	Hubei Provincial Human Organ Donation Administrative Center
18	Hunan	Hunan Provincial Human Organ Donation Administrative Center
19	Guangdong	Guangdong Red Cross Society Organ Donation Office
20	Guangxi	Guangxi Zhuang Autonomous Region Human Organ Donation Administrative Center
21	Hainan	Hainan Red Cross Medical and Donation Service Center
22	Chongqing	Chongqing Organ and Remains Donation Administrative Center
23	Sichuan	Sichuan Provincial Human Organ Donation Administrative Center
24	Guizhou	Guizhou Provincial Human Organ, Cell and Tissue Donation Administrative Center
25	Yunnan	Yunnan Provincial Human Organ Donation Administrative Center
26	Shaanxi	Shaanxi Provincial Human Organ Donation Administrative Center
27	Gansu	Gansu Red Cross Humanitarian Affairs Service Center

		Continued
No.	Provinces (Autonomous regions/ Municipalities)	Name of institutions
28	Qinghai	Qinghai Provincial Human Organ Donation Administrative Center
29	Ningxia	Ningxia Hui Autonomous Region Red Cross Disaster Preparedness and Relief Center
30	Xinjiang	Human Organ Donation Administrative Center of Xinjiang Uygur Autonomous Region

1.1.2 Coordinator team

In 2023, the China Human Organ Donation Administrative Center conducted three training sessions for national human organ donation coordinators in Harbin, Heilongjiang Province, Linyi, Shandong Province, and Wuhan, Hubei Province, training more than 400 newly recruited coordinators. There were 2 602 registered coordinators nationwide as of the conclusion of 2023, including 1 127 Red Cross staff and 1 475 Red Cross volunteers from medical institutions (Figure 1–1).

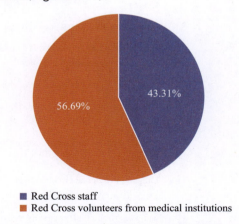

Figure 1-1　Composition of national human organ donation coordinators by the end of 2023

1.1.3 Capacity building

In 2023, the China Human Organ Donation Administrative Center held the inaugural academic lecture for human organ donation experts in Changsha, Hunan Province, with more than 300 people including relevant responsible individuals of Red Cross Societies, representatives from medical institutions and relevant (autonomous regions and municipalities) experts from all provinces participating. The 7th national advanced training course on human organ donation was held in Haikou, Hainan Province training more than 120 management personnel and core staff members. Two teacher training courses for coordinator capacity building were held in Taiyuan, Shanxi Province and Kunming, Yunnan Province, training more than 70 coordinator teachers.

1.2 Registration of human organ donation volunteers

1.2.1 Regional distribution of volunteer registration

In 2023, the number of newly registered volunteers for human organ donation nationwide was 820 000, bringing the total number of human organ donation volunteers nationwide to 6.65 million. The top ten provinces with the largest number were Guangdong (568 000), Shandong (542 900), Jiangsu (495 200), Henan (451 800), Sichuan (448 100), Zhejiang (342 100), Anhui (322 800), Hubei (274 100), Hebei (271 300), and Hunan (254 900) (Figure 1-2).

1.2.2 Volunteer registration rate per 10,000 people

By the end of 2023, the voluntary registration rate for human organ donation per 10 000 population in China was 47.2‰. The top ten provinces were Beijing (83.9), Jiangsu (58.1), Tianjin (57.3), Shaanxi (55.1), Shandong (53.6), Sichuan (53.5), Anhui (52.7), Shanghai (52.2), Zhejiang (51.6), and Jilin (50.3) (Figure 1-3).

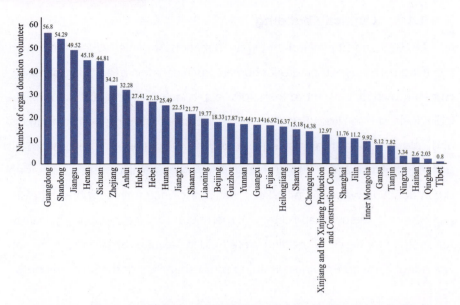

Figure 1-2 Number of voluntary registration for human organ donation in each province (autonomous region and municipality) across China by the end of 2023

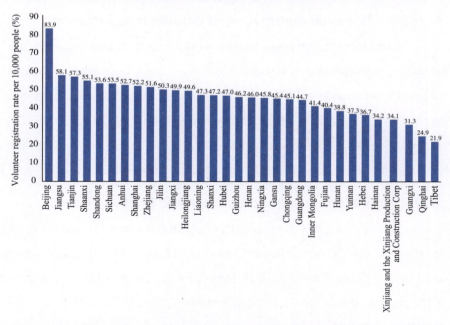

Figure 1-3 Registration rate per 10 000 population in each province (autonomous region and municipality) across China by the end of 2023

1.2.3 Age distribution of registered volunteers

The age composition of volunteer registraats for human organ donation nationwide was as follows: 40% were at the age of 18–25, 38.2% were at the age of 26–35, 14.6% were at the age of 36–45, 5.6% were at the age of 46–60, and 1.6% were older than 60 (Figure 1–4), with the majority of young and middle-aged registrants.

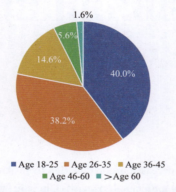

Figure 1-4　Age composition of national volunteer registrants for human organ donation by the end of 2023

1.3　Organ donation in China

1.3.1　Annual donation amount

In 2023, number of deceased donation in China was 6 454, increased by 14.39% compared to 2022. Since 2010, the cumulative number of deceased organ donations has reached over 49 000 cases, with a total of over 153 000 solid organs being donated. The top ten provinces (autonomous regions and municipalities) with the most cases of organ donation in 2023 were Guangdong (774), Shandong (669), Guangxi (561), Hubei (462), Beijing (419), Hunan (314), Henan (310), Zhejiang (283), Shaanxi (280) and Sichuan (245) (Figure 1–5).

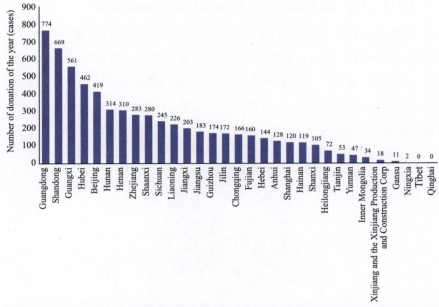

Figure 1-5 Number of deceased organ donation by province (autonomous region and municipality) across China in 2023

1.3.2 Donation rate per million population

In 2023, the organ donation rate per million population (PMP) was 4.58 nationwide. The ten provinces (autonomous regions and municipalities) with the highest PMP were Beijing (19.2), Hainan (11.4), Guangxi (11.2), Hubei (7.9), Jilin (7.4), Shaanxi (7.1), Shandong (6.6), Guangdong (6.1), Liaoning (5.4), and Chongqing (5.2) (Figure 1–6).

1.3.3 Gender composition of organ donors

In 2023, male donors accounted for the majority of deceased organ donors in China, with a proportion of 81.05%, while females accounted for 18.95% (Figure 1–7).

Chapter 1　Human Organ Donation in China

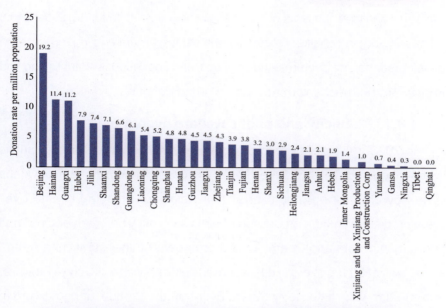

Figure 1-6　PMP of each province (autonomous region and municipality) of deceased donors across China in 2023

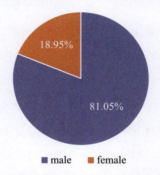

Figure 1-7　Gender composition of deceased organ donors across China in 2023

1.4　Progress of related work

In 2023, under the guidance and support of the National Health Commission and the Red Cross Society of China, the China Organ Donation Administrative Center, the China Organ Transplantation Development Foundation and other institutions have been committed to vigorously promoting the organ donation concepts publicity, voluntary registration for organ donation, witnessing organ donation processes, the establishment and implementation of volunteer service systems and activities, and continuously establishing and improving the mechanism for human organ donation.

1.4.1 Publicity and public welfare events

In 2023, multiple themed promotional activities targeting the public were conducted. The brochure "Life & Encounter" and promotional videos "The Power of One Person" and "Life Relay & Spreading Great Love" were produced, and the production of films such as "The Team of One" and "Ferryman of Life and Death" was promoted. The inaugural "Life Relay" sports event for human organ donation was held in Nanchang, Jiangxi Province, and a nationwide "Life Relay Sports Event on the Cloud" for human organ donation was initiated. Activities were carried out in the form of "Internet + sports check-in + concept popularization," attracted a total of over 436 teams and more than 49 000 participants from 31 competition areas. A three-month-long nationwide promotion campaign regarding the organ donation volunteer registry was implemented. Over 100 promotional activities for organ donation were conducted in hospitals, universities, enterprises, communities, and other venues by local Red Cross Societies under the theme of Promise of Life & transmission Great Love. At the same time, 31 themed Party Day a ctivities for the life relay were conducted; nearly 200 institutions participated in the China Organ Donation Day Thematic Campaign, resulting institations in a total popularization volume of 300 million. The Weibo topic ranked ninth on the trending list on the day. Additionally, a series of public welfare projects under the Life Relay, Hundred Cities Tour Initiative were launched in 12 cities, the concept of organ donation was promoted continuously and extensively through various forms.

1.4.2 Volunteer registration and consultation service

In 2023, there were 820 000 newly registered human organ donation volunteers, with over 24 000 consultation calls answered, more than 8 500 text message inquiries responded to, and over 1 100 consultation emails processed. More than 600 000 sets of physical card and appreciation letters were produced and distributed to registered organ donation volunteers. Efforts to expand channels for volunteer registration were continued, as the Love & Hope organ donation volunteer service system has completed technical integration with 133 cooperative institutions, providing more convenient registration channels for people with a willingness to donate.

1.4.3 Donation witness and case reports

In 2023, 6 454 cases of human organ donation witnessing were concluded. In accordance with the principles of "voluntary and unpaid", the coordinators objectively witnessed and documented the processes of willingness confirmation, procedure and results of organ procurement and allocation on site, filling in the relevant in formation of donation cases timely and accurately through the China Human Organ Donation Case Reporting Management System, protecting the rights and interests of donors and their families.

1.4.4 Commemoration and humanitarian care

A month-long nationwide commemorative event for human organ donation themed "Life & Encounter" was initiated. The 2023 National Commemorative and Publicity Event for Human Organ Donation was held in Changsha, Hunan Province, with a synchronized online commemorative event organized to honor the selfless dedication of donors and their families. 29 new commemorative venues were established in Yangquan, Shanxi Province, Yueqing, Zhejiang Province, Shantou, Guangdong Province and other places. Donation certificates, commemorative medals, and condolence letters were issued to each family of human organ donors, and various care activities such as follow-up visits, condolences, psychological comfort, and education assistance for children were widely conducted. Charitable organizations such as the China Organ Transplantation Development Foundation fulfilled their missions and responsibilities, rallying social attention and providing charitable assistance to families facing financial difficulties, aiming at fostering an atmosphere of solidarity and mutual assistance throughout society, and cultivating a culture and social environment that support organ donation and are in line with China's national conditions.

1.4.5 Development of volunteer service system

A seminar on volunteer services for human organ donation and literary and artistic creation was conducted, alongside preparations for the formation of the China Human Organ Donation Volunteer Service Working Committee. A month-long nationwide volunteer initiative focused on human organ donation was launched, facilitating the execution of 10 volunteer service projects, including "Little Orange Lamp" and "Angel Loves Mom". By the end of 2023, over 600 volunteer service teams for human organ donation had been established nationwide, comprising more than 20 000 volunteers. The National Youth Volunteer Service Corps for Organ Donation in the Health Sector was launched, enlisting volunteers from the health sector, universities, and other organ donation related organizations across the nation to promote the advancement of organ donation in China through tangible efforts.

1.4.6 Construction of communication and information platform

12 issues of the *China Human Organ Donation Work Newsletter* were compiled and distributed to more than 700 institutions and individuals nationwide. By the end of 2023, the WeChat official account "China Human

Organ Donation" boasted more than 5.3 million followers. Newly launched platforms include the "China Human Organ Donation" Alipay Lifestyle account and Himalaya FM podcast account. The official website and micro-website of the China Human Organ Donation Administrative Center have been redesigned and upgraded, along with the volunteer registration and case reporting management system for human organ donation. The China Organ Transplantation Development Foundation's social media network amassed over 1.655 million followers. Monthly reports were disseminated to 132 collaborating units for organ donation volunteer services, aligning statistical data on work progress. The integration with the China Organ Transplant Response System (COTRS) has been finalized, facilitating the automatic verification of volunteer registration data for potential organ donors.

1.5 Future outlook

Comprehensively implement the *Regulations on Human Organ Donation and Transplantation*, and plan to formulate and issue related supporting documents regarding donation witnessing and humanitarian care. Persist in advancing the formulation of regulations, systems, and operational mechanisms for human organ donation, while continuously improving the legalization, professionalization, and standardization of organ donation practices. Enhance the construction, management, and service of coordinator teams, and furnish more substantial support for their daily operations. Conduct publicity events, assist local organizations in organizing various promotional activities, and advocate for human organ donation in hospitals, universities, communities, and enterprises.

Continue to broaden the channels for organ donation volunteer registration. Promote the establishment of commemorative facilities for donors in cities higher than the county level that have the capacity, support provincial–level Red Cross Societies in establishing and enhancing humanitarian care working mechanisms, thus further foster a social environment that supports the selfless dedication spirit of organ donation.

Chapter 2 Donated Organ Procurement in China

Data scope

The data presented in this Chapter is sourced from the basic information database of Organ Procurement Organization (OPO) and the China Organ Transplant Response System (COTRS). It encompasses information regarding the organizational structure of OPO, team building, and human organ procurement. The statistical period was from January 1st, 2023 to December 31st, 2023.

Statistical methods

Data in this chapter were all analyzed with descriptive statistical methods.

Chapter highlights

(1) By the end of 2023, there were a total of 109 OPOs in China, with 1 261 staff members nationwide, averaging 12 staff members per OPO.

(2) In 2023, 20 OPOs across the nation recorded an annual donation volume of 100 cases or more, representing 53.24% of the total annual donations in China.

(3) The proportion of organ donors from brain death significantly increased year by year. The utilization rate of procured organs has slightly

decreased compared to 2022, while the number of organs procured per donor has increased. The incidence rates of primary nonfunction (PNF) and delayed graft function (DGF) following organ transplantation have maintained a favorable level.

(4) In the future, the construction of OPO as a specific discipline of hospital should be further strengthened, training programs targeted at the donor hospitals should be comprehensively promoted, and capacity on donated organ procurement should be continuously enhanced. At the meantime, evaluation on capacity of organ donation and procurement should be initiated to establish a new development paradigm for organ donation in the health sector.

2.1 Development and construction of human donated organ procurement system

On March 1st, 2014, led by the State Council, the China Human Organ Donation and Transplantation Committee was established. The Five Major Systems, which includes the human organ donation system, human organ procurement and allocation system, human organ transplantation clinical service system, human organ procurement and transplantation quality control system, as well as the supervision system for organ donation and transplantation have been launched. The China Human Organ Donation and Transplantation Committee coordinates and oversees the systems.

From the perspective of Five Major Systems, donated organ procurement is a vital procedure which connects organ donation with allocation, as well as encompasses all essential processes from donation to transplantation. This procedure is primarily carried out by the Organ Procurement Organization (OPO), which consists of coordinators, physicians, nurses, data reporters, and administrators. Responsibilities of OPO include public education, identification and referral of potential organ donors, emergency care, maintenance and evaluation of donors, applying for death determination, assistance with ethic review process, donated organ procurement, and post-donation restoration.

In 2015, China has undergone a thorough transformation to donation from deceased citizens, ushering in a new era with continuous and healthy development. Since 2016, China has consistently ranked second globally and first in Asia in terms of number of deceased donations. From 2015 to 2023, and donated more than 140 200 solid organs. China has completed a total of 46 700 cases of organ donation.

On December 14th, 2023, the *Regulations on Human Organ Donation and Transplantation* (hereinafter referred to as the *Regulations*) were issued, emphasizing the significance of organ donation, enhancing commendation and guidance for organ donation, and anticipated to serve as a catalyst for the high-quality and sustainable development of organ donation and transplantation in China. The *Regulations* delineated comprehensive management protocols for organ procurement and allocation, elucidated the supervisory responsibilities of provincial health authorities, specified the criteria for medical institutions involved in cadaveric organ procurement, and outlined the pertinent requirements for medical institutions to report information related to organ donors. The *Regulations* delineated the fundamental prerequisites for medical institutions seeking involvement in organ procurement, stipulated financial management criteria for organ procurement processes, and established quality control standards. It also proposed mandates for hospitals to perform medical evaluations of donors and donated organs, as well as risk assessments for transplantation.

In 2023, in accordance with the relevent requirements of the National Health Commission, the National Quality Control Center for Donated Organ

Procurement (OPQC) has vigorously improved the quality control system for human donated organ procurement through the construction of a three-tier quality control network. It has undertaken specialized investigations under the "Quality Improvement Initiative for Organ Procurement" to perpetually advance standardized management and capacity augmentation of OPOs. Additionally, it has initiated the train-the-trainer program on enhancing the capability of organ donation, with an aim of comprehensively promoting organ donation related work in secondary and above-level medical institutions.

2.2 Distribution and construction of OPOs

2.2.1 Distribution of OPOs

By the end of 2023, there were 109 OPOs across China, one of which was a provincial unified OPO with an independent legal entity, six of which were provincial unified OPOs affiliated with medical institutions, 22 of which were joint OPOs, and 80 of which were established within medical institutions (Figure 2-1). Provinces (autonomous regions and municipalities) that have built provincial unified OPOs were Shanxi, Jilin, Tianjin, Hainan, Zhejiang, Jiangsu, Yunnan; provinces (autonomous regions and municipalities) that have established joint OPO working mechanisms were Guangdong, Beijing, Hunan, Shanghai, Hebei, Fujian, and Heilongjiang.

2.2.2 Team building

Having an adequate staff complement is a prerequisite for ensuring the success of human organ procurement. According to the OPO basic information database, in 2023, there were 1 261 staff members involved in human organ procurement, averaging 12 staff per OPO. Among them, 29.63% of OPOs had fewer than six staff members, 44.44% had between 6 and 12, and 25.93% had more than 12 staff members.

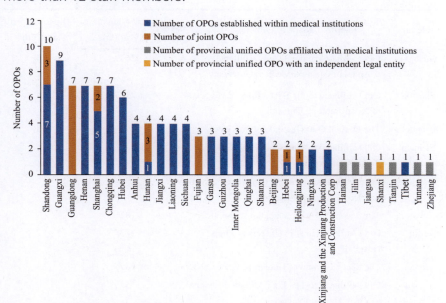

Figure 2-1   Number of OPOs by provinces (autonomous regions and municipalities) and the organizational structure across China in 2023

2.3   Organ donation in China

2.3.1   Overall situation

In 2023, 20 OPOs achieved more than 100 cases of deceased donation, accounted for 53.24% of the total number of deceased donations in China (Table 2-1).

Table 2-1   Top 20 OPOs by number of donations in 2023

Region	Name of OPO	Number of donations of the year (Case)	Organizational structure*
Zhejiang	Zhejiang Provincial Human Organ Procurement Service Management Center	283	2
Beijing	Joint OPO of the Northern Part, Beijing City	275	3

Report on Organ Donation and Transplantation in China (2023)

Continued

Region	Name of OPO	Number of donations of the year (Case)	Organizational structure*
Guangxi	OPO affiliated to the Second Affiliated Hospital of Guangxi Medical University	267	4
Shaanxi	OPO affiliated to the First Affiliated Hospital of Xi'an Jiaotong University	238	4
Guangdong	The First OPO of Guangdong Province	194	3
Sichuan	OPO affiliated to West China Hospital of Sichuan University	194	4
Jiangsu	Jiangsu Provincial Human Organ Procurement Service Management Center	183	2
Guangdong	The Second OPO of Guangdong Province	182	3
Jilin	OPO Affiliated to Jilin University First Hospital	172	2
Hunan	The Second Group of Hunan Province OPO	162	3
Henan	OPO affiliated to The First Affiliated Hospital of Zhengzhou University	158	4
Beijing	Joint OPO of the Southern Part, Beijing City	144	3
Shandong	Joint OPO affiliated to the Affiliated Hospital of Qingdao University	141	3
Hubei	OPO affiliated to Zhongnan Hospital of Wuhan University	140	4
Hebei	The Second Working Group of Hebei Provincial OPO	136	3
Hubei	OPO affiliated to Tongji Hospital Affiliated to Tongji Medical College of Huazhong University of Science &Technology	134	4
Hainan	Hainan Provincial OPO	119	2
Shandong	OPO affiliated to Shandong Provincial Qianfoshan Hospital	107	4
Shanxi	Shanxi Provincial Human Organ Procurement and Allocation Service Center	105	1
Liaoning	OPO affiliated to General Hospital of Northern Theater Command of PLA	102	4

Note: Organizational Structure: 1. Provincial unified OPO (independent legal entity); 2. Provincial unified OPO (affiliated to medical institutions); 3. Joint OPO; 4. Traditional OPO established within medical institutions.

2.3.2 Proportion of different organ donation types

In 2023, 70.70% of deceased donors (DDs) were donor after brain death (DBD), 21.71% of DDs were donors after circulatory death (DCD), 7.59% of DDs were donor after brain and circulatory death (DBCD) (Figure 2-2). Proportion of DBD was 3.96 percentage points higher than that of 2022.

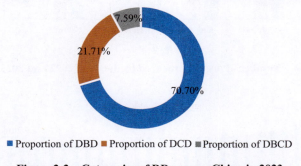

Figure 2-2　Categories of DDs across China in 2023

2.4　Procurement and utilization of organs

In 2023, 20 854 donated organs from deceased donors were procured by Organ Procurement Organizations (OPOs) across China, an increase of 15.71% compared to 2022. The number of organs procured per donor was 3.23, representing a certain improvement over 2022. Specifically, the number of livers, kidneys, heart, and lungs procured per donor was 0.92, 1.87, 0.16, and 0.28, respectively. Compared to 2022 number (0.93 for livers and 1.88 for kidneys), there was a slight decline in the number of livers and kidneys procured per donor. However, the number of hearts and lungs procured per donor increased to 0.16 and 0.28, respectively, from 0.13 and 0.26 in 2022 (Figure 2-3). Nine provinces (autonomous regions and municipalities) exceeded the national average in terms of the number of organs procured per donor (Figure 2-4).

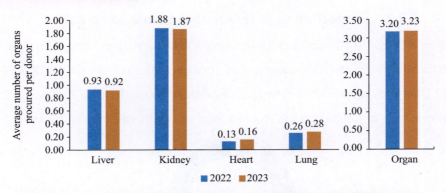

Figure 2-3 Number of organs procured by donor of 2022 and 2023 in China

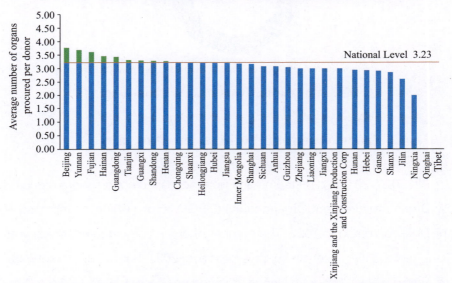

Figure 2-4 Average number of organs procured per donor by province (autonomous region and municipality) in 2023

In 2023, the national average utilization rate of donated organs was 96.55%, which was lower than that of 2022 (96.74%). Utilization rate of livers was 95.99%, that of kidneys was 96.84%, that of hearts was 96.10%, and that of lungs was 96.71% (Figure 2-5). Utilization rate of donated organs of 14 provinces (autonomous regions and municipalities) surpassed national level. Utilization rate of organs of Inner Mongolia, Gansu and Ningxia were 100% (Figure 2-6).

Chapter 2 Donated Organ Procurement in China

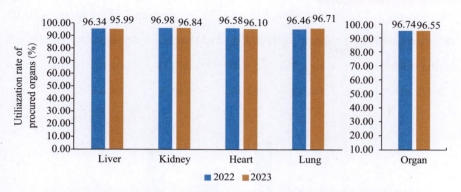

Figure 2-5 Utilization rate of organs procured in China in 2022 and 2023

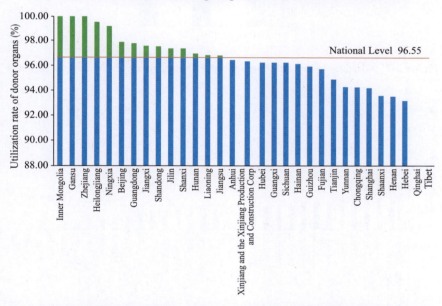

Figure 2-6 Utilization rate of donor organs of each province (autonomous region and municipality) across China in 2023

2.5 Quality of donor organs

2.5.1 Incidence rate of primary graft non-function (PNF) of donor organs

In 2023, the incidence rate of primary graft non–function (PNF) of donor

123

organs was 1.20%, higher than that of 2022, lower than 2021 (Figure 2–7). 10 provinces (autonomous regions and municipalities) surpassed national level (Figure 2–8).

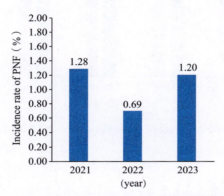

Figure 2-7　Changes in the incidence rate of PNF in China over the past three years

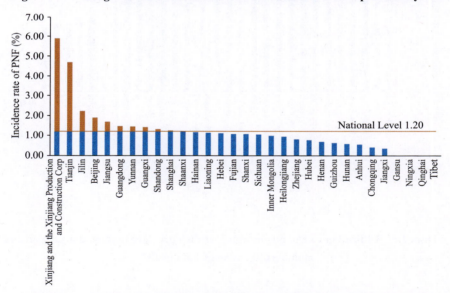

Figure 2-8　Incidence rate of PNF of each province (autonomous region and municipality) of China in 2023

2.5.2　Incidence rate of delayed graft function (DGF) of donor organs

In 2023, the incidence rate of delayed graft function (DGF) was 10.25%, higher

Chapter 2 Donated Organ Procurement in China

than that of 2022 (Figure 2-9). The incidence of DGF in 10 provinces (autonomous regions and municipalities) surpassed the national average level (Figure 2-10).

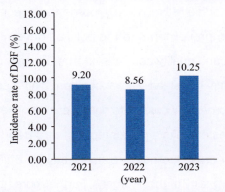

Figure 2-9 Changes in the incidence rate of DGF in China in the pasr three years

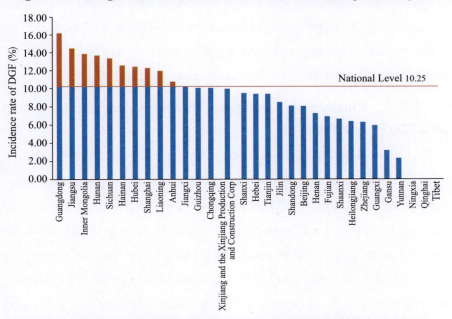

Figure 2-10 Incidence rate of DGF of each province (autonomous region and municipality) of China in 2023

2.6 Features and future outlook

Under the leadership and support of the National Health Commission of the People's Republic of China and the China Human Organ Donation and Transplantation Committee, the "Chinese model" of organ donation and transplantation has achieved rapid development. Especially in recent years, with the ongoing improvements to the policies governing organ donation and transplantation and quality control systems, China's organ donation and transplantation industry has steadily advanced from high-speed development to high-quality development. According to data, it can be observed that the annual volume of donations exhibits a consistent upward trend. Concurrently, the generation of donor organs remains relatively stable, while there is a gradual improvement in the quality of these organs. Furthermore, there is an enhanced prognosis associated with organ transplantation from donors, and the technical capabilities of OPOs are continuously advancing. As a large country with 1.4 billion population, management and quality control on organ procurement will continue to develop from the following four aspects.

2.6.1 Consistently strengthen the disciplinary construction of OPOs in hospitals

In accordance with the relevant *Regulations* requirements, when advancing the disciplinary construction of OPOs in hospitals, the high-quality development principle should be followed, an innovative model should be maintained, and a scientific management concept based on precise quality control should be retained. Efforts should be focused on refining the organizational structure of OPOs, upgrading the working environment and necessary facilities regarding donated organ procurement, enhancing capabilities of personnels, establishing a long-term management mechanism, strictly implementing core medical regulations, developing clinical protocols for organ procurement, and conducting scientific organ maintenance, donated organ quality assessment and quality control. The special investigation named Quality Improvement Initiatives in Organ Procurement should be continuously conducted, with an aim of carrying out targeted quality control in a problem-oriented way. Efforts should be made on advancing the implementation of standardized procedures and technical specifications for human organ procurement, discussing the challenges of homogeneous management under different organizational forms, and proposing reasonable suggestions for improvement.

2.6.2 Comprehensively promote the Donor Hospital Training Program

To enhance awareness of pertinent policies and regulations regarding human organ procurement and to improve the technical competencies of medical personnel at institutions that produce organ donors, all regions should be encouraged to actively organize Donor Hospital Training Programs and to promote and implement the *Regulations*. The OPQC is tasked with executing train-the-trainer programs and establishing a trainer pool, whereas each OPO is responsible for developing its own training programs and plans, conducting Donor Hospital Training Courses for medical institutions in their service areas as necessary, thereby perpetually enhancing regional PMP.

2.6.3 Promote the continuous enhancement of human organ procurement capabilities

Efforts should focus on augmenting the organ procurement capabilities of OPOs, enforcing ethical review requirements for organ donation, advancing microbial infection gene sequencing of donors, conducting pathogen culture and microbial gene sequencing of organ preservation solutions, ensuring pathological biopsies of donated organs, and enhancing clinical translational research aimed at optimizing the quality of donated organs. The employment of particular technologies, including extracorporeal membrane oxygenation (ECMO) and mechanical perfusion, should be promoted to enhance the quality of donated organs.

2.6.4 Initiate the evaluation work regarding organ donation and procurement capabilities

Capacity assessments aimed at OPOs for organ procurement should be performed to continually enhance the development and administration of OPOs. This type of evaluation should be extended to secondary–level medical institutions and higher within the service area of a specific OPO, and records for organ donation should be created to monitor organ donations from these hospitals and enhance the quality of donated organs. Organ donation in medical institutions at the secondary level and above should be significantly promoted to establish a new paradigm for the advancement of organ donation within the nation's healthcare sector.

Chapter 3 Human Organ Allocation and Sharing in China

Data scope

Data showed in this chapter are mainly based on data from the China Organ Transplant Response System (COTRS), spanning from January 1st, 2015, to December 31st, 2023.

Statistical methods

Descriptive statistical analysis was employed to analyze the basic information of organ donors and patients waiting for organ transplantation.

Chapter highlights

(1) In 2023, 10 778 human organ donations were completed in China, including 6 454 cases (59.88%) of cadaveric organ donations and 4 324 cases (40.12%) of living related donations. A total of 23 905 organ transplantation surgeries were performed, with 19 581 cases (81.91%) from cadaveric organ donations and 4 324 cases (18.09%) from living related organ donations, including 119 cases of combined multiple organ transplantation. During the same period, 160 767 people were waiting for organ transplantation.

(2) In 2023, the median age of DDs in China was 49. The number of pediatric donations (donors below the age of 18) was 478, accounting for 7.41% of the total. In terms of donation classifications, 70.70% were

donations from brain-dead individuals. Cerebrovascular accidents were the primary cause of death, accounting for 53.59%.

(3) In 2023, there were 160 767 patients waiting for organ transplantation, including 134 011 waiting for kidney transplantation, 21 940 waiting for liver transplantation, 3 182 waiting for heart transplantation, and 1 634 waiting for lung transplantation. At the end of 2023, 45 212 individuals were no longer waiting for organ transplantation, while 115 555 patients with organ failure were still awaiting, among whom the number of patients waiting for kidney, liver, heart, and lung transplantation were 105 458, 8 288, 1 457, and 352 respectively.

A total of 46 688 cases of deceased donation (DD) have been completed in China from January 1st, 2015 to December 31st, 2023. PMP increased from 2.01 in 2015 to 4.58 in 2023. In 2023, 10 778 human organ donations were completed in China, including 6 454 cases (59.88%) of cadaveric organ donations and 4 324 cases (40.12%) of living related donations A total of 23 905 organ transplantation surgeries were performed, with 19 581 cases (81.91%) from cadaveric organ donations and 4 324 cases (18.09%) from living related organ donations, including 119 cases of combined multiple organ transplantation.

Since the implementation of the *Regulations on Human Organ Transplantation* in 2007, it has played a crucial role in promoting the fair allocation of human organs. China has initially established a system for the procurement and allocation of human organs that complies with international principles such as the *Guiding Principles on Human Cell, Tissue and Organ Transplantation* of the World Health Organization. In 2013, the China Organ Transplant Response System (COTRS) was launched for automatic allocation of cadaveric donated organs, effectively ensuring scientific, fair, impartial,

Chapter 3 Human Organ Allocation and Sharing in China

and transparent organ allocation. In 2018, the National Health Commission of the People's Republic of China (NHC) issued the Notice on Issuing the Basic Principles and Core Policies for the Allocation and Sharing of Human Organs in China, which revised the *Notice of the Ministry of Health on Issuing the Basic Principles and Core Policies for the Allocation and Sharing of Human Organs for Liver and Kidney Transplantation* (MOH–BMA〔2010〕No. 113), and officially developed the core policies for the allocation and sharing of hearts and lungs. These combined formulated the *Basic Principles and Core Policies for the Allocation and Sharing of Human Organs in China* (Hereinafter referred to as the *Core Policy of Organ Allocation*).

In 2023, the newly revised *Regulations on Human Organ Donation and Transplantation* elevated the relevant provisions on the procurement and allocation management of human organs from departmental normative documents to administrative regulations, providing a legal foundation for the management of human organ procurement and allocation. The organ procurement and allocation system will inevitably become increasingly regulated, professionalized, and scientific. Organ donation and transplantation will inevitably evolve to be more equitable, sustainable, and of higher quality, thereby further protecting health and interests of the people.

COTRS is an essential part of China's organ donation and transplantation system, which consists of "potential organ donor identification system" "human organ donor registration and organ matching system" "human organ transplant waiting list system" and the regulatory platform. As a highly specialized information system, COTRS is responsible for implementing the relevant laws, regulations, and scientific policies of organ allocation and sharing in China. It enforces the national policy for scientific organ allocation, enables automatic organ allocation and sharing, provides monitoring on national and local regulatory agencies, ensures the traceability of organ procurement and allocation, minimizes human interference, and guarantees the fair, just, and open allocation of donor organs. These measures are a cornerstone to build trust of the Chinese citizens in the process of organ donation after death.

3.1 Distribution of transplant hospitals in China

As of December 31st, 2023, there were 188 medical institutions qualified for organ transplantation in China, an increase of 5 compared to 2022. The distribution of these institutions by province (autonomous region and municipality) is shown in Figure 3-1. The ten provinces (autonomous regions and municipalities) with the greatest number of transplant hospitals were Guangdong (21), Beijing (17), Shanghai (13), Shandong (12), Fujian (10), Hunan (10), Zhejiang (10), Hubei (8), Henan (7), and Jiangsu (7).

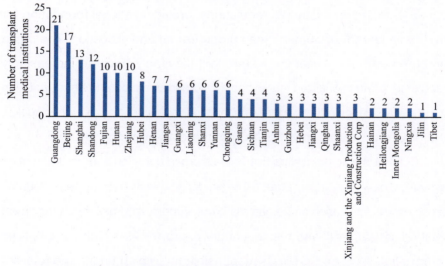

Figure 3-1 Distribution of transplant medical institutions of each province (autonomous region and municipality) of China in 2023

Chapter 3 Human Organ Allocation and Sharing in China

3.2 Overview of human organ donation

3.2.1 Number of human organ donation

From 2015 to 2023, the number of deceased organ donations and the PMP in China have steadily increased, rising from 2 766 cases in 2015 to 6 454 cases in 2023, and the PMP has increased from 2.01 in 2015 to 4.58 in 2023 (Figure 3–2). Between 2020 and 2023, the number of deceased organ donation in China has maintained a steady growth (Figure 3–3).

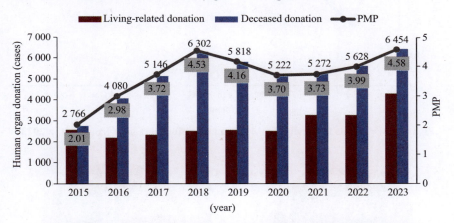

Figure 3-2 Number of organ donations in China from 2015 to 2023

Note: Data of population from 2015 to 2019 is obtained from the China Health Statistics Yearbook. Data of population from 2020 to 2023 is obtained from National Bureau of Statistics of China.

3.2.2 Features of deceased donors

In 2023, the median age of DDs in China was 49. The number of pediatric donations (donors below the age of 18) was 478, accounting for 7.41% of the total. Among them, 87 donors (18.20%) were under the age of 2, 103 donors (21.55%) were 2-6 years old, 132 (27.62%) were donors aged 7-13, and 156 (32.64%) were donors aged 14-18. The majority of donors was male (81.05%). The dominating blood type of the donors was Type O (37.08%), followed by Type A and Type B, each accounting for 28.60% and 25.98% of all donors. Type

AB accounted for 8.34% (Figure 3-4). 70.70% of DDs were C- I (DBD), 21.71% of DDs were C- II (DCD), and 7.59% of DDs were C- III (DBCD) (Figure 3-5).

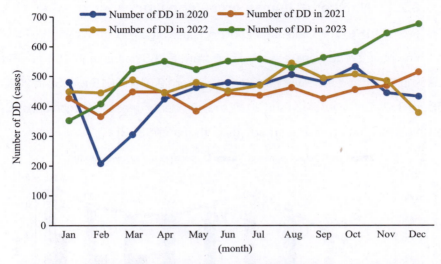

Figure 3-3　Trends in the number of organ donations in China from 2020 to 2023

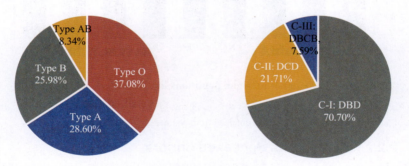

Figure 3-4　Distribution of blood types of DDs of China in 2023

Figure 3-5　Categories of DDs of China in 2023

From 2015 to 2023, trauma and cerebrovascular accidents were two of the major causes of donors' death, accounting for 86.85% of all deaths (Figure 3-6). The proportion of donors with cerebrovascular accidents had been increasing each year. From 2019, cerebrovascular accidents have overtaken trauma as the leading cause of death in DDs in China (Figure 3-7).

Chapter 3　Human Organ Allocation and Sharing in China

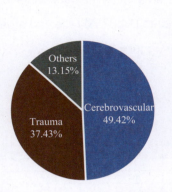

Figure 3-6　Causes of death of DDs from 2015 to 2023

Figure 3-7　Proportion of DDs death caused by cerebrovascular accidents from 2015 to 2023

3.3　Patients waiting for organ transplantation

3.3.1　Number of patients waiting for organ transplantation

From 2015 to 2023, the number of patients waiting for liver and kidney transplantation had been increasing each year (Figure 3–8). In 2023, there were 160 767 patients of organ failure waiting for organ transplantation, including 134 011 waiting for kidney transplantation, 21 940 waiting for liver transplantation, 3 182 waiting for heart transplantation, and 1 634 waiting for lung transplantation. At present, China has not established a unified national

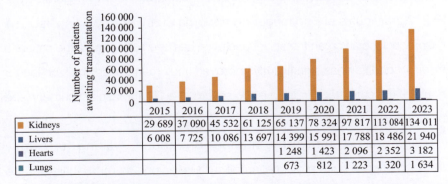

Figure 3-8　Number of patients waiting for organ transplantation from 2015 to 2023

135

registry for the patients waiting for pancreas and small intestine transplantation. During the same period, a total of 23 905 patients (14.87%) received organ transplantation surgeries across the country (Figure 3-9).

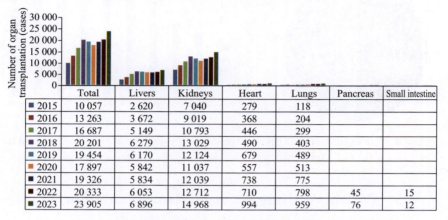

	Total	Livers	Kidneys	Heart	Lungs	Pancreas	Small intestine
2015	10 057	2 620	7 040	279	118		
2016	13 263	3 672	9 019	368	204		
2017	16 687	5 149	10 793	446	299		
2018	20 201	6 279	13 029	490	403		
2019	19 454	6 170	12 124	679	489		
2020	17 897	5 842	11 037	557	513		
2021	19 326	5 834	12 039	738	775		
2022	20 333	6 053	12 712	710	798	45	15
2023	23 905	6 896	14 968	994	959	76	12

Figure 3-9 Number of organ transplant cases from 2015 to 2023

Note: From 2015-2023, there were 8, 52, 60, 89, and 119 cases of combined multiple organs transplantation involved, respectively

3.3.2 Number of patients waiting for transplantation at the end of the year

By the end of 2023, there were still 115 555 patients waiting for transplantation surgeries, including 105 458 patients waiting for kidney transplantation, 8 288 patients waiting for liver transplantation, 1 457 and 352 patients waiting for heart and lung transplantation, respectively (Figure 3-10). 45 212 individuals are no longer on the organ transplant waiting list. The reasons include an organ transplant operation has been performed, the patient's physical condition has significantly improved and organ transplant is no longer required, the patient's condition is too severe to accept transplant surgery ,and the patient has died.

Figure 3-11 shows the number of patients waiting for kidney transplantation in each province (autonomous region and municipality) at the end of 2023. The top ten provinces (autonomous regions and municipalities)

were Zhejiang (13 322), Guangdong (13 314), Hunan (8 837), Henan (8 136), Sichuan (7 665), Shanghai (6 921), Hubei (6 038), Guangxi (5 439), Shandong (3 589), and Beijing (3 401).

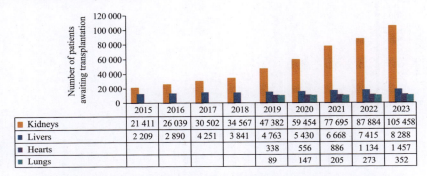

Figure 3-10 Number of patients waiting for organ transplantation at the end of each year from 2015 to 2023

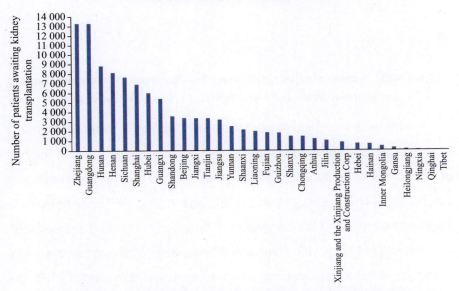

Figure 3-11 Number of patients waiting for kidney transplantation in each province (autonomous region and municipality) of China at the end of 2023

Figure 3–12 shows the number of patients waiting for liver transplantation in each province (autonomous region and municipality) of China. The top ten provinces (autonomous regions and municipalities) were Sichuan (1 775),

Guangdong (1 032), Zhejiang (748), Beijing (594), Tianjin (488), Shanghai (477), Jiangsu (421), Hubei (397), Hunan (341) and Yunnan (320).

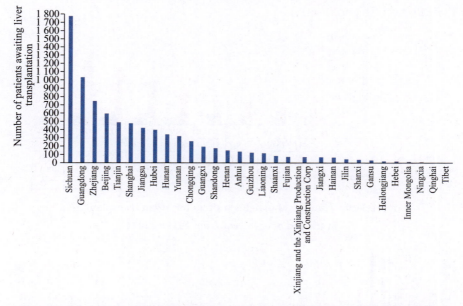

Figure 3-12   Number of patients waiting for liver transplantation in each province (autonomous region and municipality) of China at the end of 2023

Figure 3-13 shows the number of patients waiting for heart transplantation in each province (autonomous region and municipality) of China at the end of 2023. The top ten provinces (autonomous regions and municipalities) were Beijing (339), Hubei (281), Henan (142), Guangdong (107), Shanghai (97), Zhejiang (91), Hunan (72), Shaanxi (52), Shandong (41) , and Sichuan (38).

Figure 3-14 shows the number of patients waiting for lung transplantation in each province (autonomous region and municipality) at the end of 2023. The top ten provinces (autonomous regions and municipalities) were Zhejiang (82), Hubei (53), Guangdong (52), Henan (44), Anhui (18), Hunan (18), Sichuan (18), Shaanxi (11), Shanghai (11), Beijing (9) and Jiangsu (9).

Chapter 3　Human Organ Allocation and Sharing in China

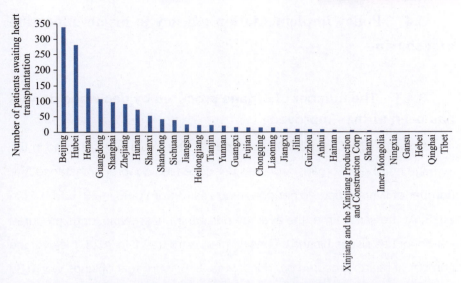

Figure 3-13　Number of patients waiting for heart transplantation in each province (autonomous region and municipality) of China at the end of 2023

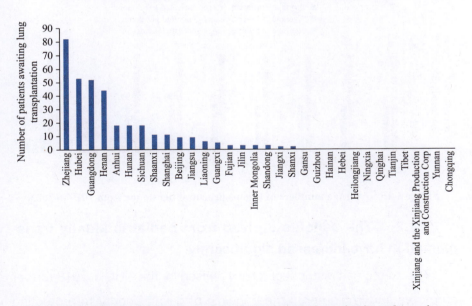

Figure 3-14　Number of patients waiting for lung transplantation in each province (autonomous region and municipality) of China at the end of 2023

3.4 Policy implementation efficacy in organ allocation and sharing

3.4.1 The number of organs procured by deceased donors has been further improved

Between 2015 and 2023, there was a discernible upward trend in the average number of organs procured per deceased donor. For instance, the number of livers procured per donor increased from 0.88 in 2015 to 0.92 in 2023. At the same time, the average number of hearts and lungs procured per donor has also exhibited a consistent upward trend. In 2023, the average number of hearts procured per donor was 0.16, while that of lungs was 0.28 (Figure 3–15).

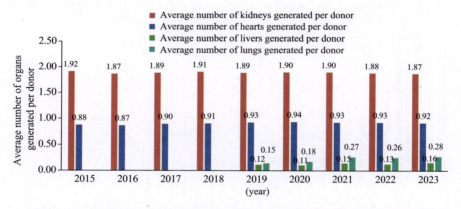

Figure 3-15 Average numbers of organs procured per donor from 2015 to 2023

3.4.2 The benefits derived from pediatric kidney transplantation have increased significantly

The core organ distribution policy revised by the NHC in 2018 further promotes and implements the principle of giving priority to protecting children's interests and promoting the allocation of public resources to children. Considering the serious adverse effects of kidney disease and dialysis treatment on the growth and development of children, kidneys from donors under the age of 18 are allocated to kidney transplant waiters under 18 in priority nationwide, increasing the chance of getting donor kidney among children waiting for transplantation.

A comparison of pediatric kidney transplantation before and after the revision of the core policies for organ allocation reveals a clear upward trend in the proportion of children among kidney transplant waiting list recipients who receive organ allocation after the implementation of the new policies. In 2023, the proportions of children and adults on the kidney transplant waiting list who received organ allocation were 31.22% and 8.29% respectively. The proportion of children receiving organ allocation was 3.8 times that of adults, indicating a significant benefit for children waiting for kidney transplants.

3.4.3 Implementation of the Green Channel Policy has facilitated organ sharing

On May 6th, 2016, the then National Health and Family Planning Commission, and other five ministries jointly issued the Notice Regarding the Establishment of a *Green Channel for the Transport of Donor Organs* (hereinafter referred to as the *Green Channel Policy*) to establish a green pathway for transportation of donor organs. The *Green Channel Policy* clarifies the responsibilities of all parties to ensure the smooth transit of donor organs and minimize the impact of transit on the quality and safety of organ transplantation.

The *Green Channel Policy* categorized organ transit into general and emergency processes based on the specific situations to achieve a fast custom clearance and priority transportation of don organs, so as to improve the efficiency and safety of organ transit, as well as reduce the waste of organs caused by transportation.

Report on Organ Donation and Transplantation in China (2023)

A comparison of the sharing of human donated organs in China before and after the implementation of the green channel policy for the transportation of human donated organs showed that in 2023, after the policy was implemented, the proportions of intra-provincial sharing and national sharing of organs increased by 8.4% and 2.0% respectively compared to the level before the policy implementation (Table 3-1).

Table 3-1 Organ sharing in China before and after the implementation of the *Green Channel Policy*

Shared Scope	Proportion of Organ Sharing at different time periods (%)			
	Before the Green Channel Policy	2022	2023	Change (between 2023 and the level before the policy implementation)
Within OPO	75.0	64.2	64.6	−10.4
Provincial-level sharing	12.6	20.6	21.0	8.4▲
National-level sharing	12.4	15.1	14.4	2.0▲

Note: ▲ indicates increases.

3.5 Feature and future outlook

Organ transplantation is a great achievement in the development of human medicine, saving lives of countless patients with end-stage diseases. In 2023, the number of organ donation and transplantation in China ranks the second in the world. COTRS plays an important role in implementing the national-level scientific allocation policies to ensure the fairness, justice and openness of organ distribution in China.

3.5.1 The work of human organ donation has been proceeding smoothly and orderly, with efficient and standardized allocation processes

In 2023, there were 6 454 cases of organ donation from deceased donors nationwide, 3.25 organs were recovered per donor, and utilization rate of all organs was 96.33%. The number of human organ donations has reached an all-time high, while the organ donation process was stable and organized, and the allocation process was efficient and standardized. In the meantime, only 23 905 of the approximately 160 800 patients waiting for organ transplantation in China received transplant surgery. Organ deficiency continues to be the primary factor inhibiting the development of organ transplantation. In the future, continued efforts should be made to increase the promotion of organ donation, enhance the efficacy of promotion, and increase the number of organ donations.

3.5.2 Ensure scientific and fair allocation, and promote the legalization of human organ allocation

The amended *Regulations* explicitly state that "cadaveric organs shall be allocated uniformly via the allocation system established by the health department of the State Council", and that "medical institutions involved in the procurement and transplantation of cadaveric organs must accurately complete and update pertinent medical data of cadaveric organ donors and patients applying for organ transplantations in the allocation system, and must not falsify or alter data". It mandates that "medical institutions and their personnel must implement the allocation outcomes from the allocation system" and shall not "conduct human organ transplantation utilizing cadaveric organs that have not been allocated via the allocation system or human organs of indeterminate origin". This set of regulations establishes explicit standards and criteria for the organ allocation process, essential components, and the implementation of allocation outcomes.

Moreover, the Regulations delineate explicit boundaries for the distribution of cadaveric organs, establishing a legal framework to combat illicit activities and protect the rightful entitlements of donors and patients on transplant waiting lists. This facilitates the standardization of organ allocation and fosters the healthy and sustainable advancement of organ donation and transplantation in China. The *Regulations* mandate that "the health department of the State Council shall regularly disclose the status of cadaveric organ donation and allocation", fostering social oversight, improving public awareness regarding organ donation and transplantation, and promoting increased participation in cadaveric organ donation to benefit more patients.

3.5.3 Revisions to the national policy on human organ allocation and sharing should be conducted

Aiming at carrying out the education campaign on the study and implementation of the Thought on Socialism with Chinese Characteristics for a New Era, especially at promoting in-depth investigation and research, thus enhance the scientific and advanced nature of organ allocation policies in China, and facilitate the high-quality development of organ donation and transplantation in China, the COTRS Scientific Committee will continuously conduct research activities on the national policy of human organ allocation and sharing, jointly exploring clinical needs and policy recommendations for human organ donation and transplantation.

Chapter 4 Liver Transplantation in China

Data scope

Data showed in this chapter are mainly based on data from the China Liver Transplant Registry (CLTR), spanning from January 1st, 2015, to December 31st, 2023.

Statistical methods

Descriptive statistical analysis was used to summarize the basic characteristics of liver transplant recipients, and survival analysis was conducted using the Kaplan-Meier method.

Chapter highlights

(1) In 2023, the number of liver transplants in China reached a historical high. A total of 6 896 liver transplantation surgeries were performed, representing a 13.9% increase compared to 2022; in 2023, 12 medical institutions performed 150 or more liver transplantation surgeries, accounting for 42.9% of the total number; by the end of 2023, the number of medical institutions qualified for liver transplantation had reached 118.

(2) The mean cold ischemia time, mean length of anhepatic phase, mean intraoperative blood loss, and mean volume of red blood cell (RBC) transfusion during operation and mean surgery time, which are overall quality indicators of liver transplantation in China, have shown an trend of

improvement year by year.

(3) Pediatric liver transplantation in China has been steadily developing, source of donor livers have been actively expanded, and medical quality and service levels of liver transplantation have been continuously improved.

4.1 Distribution of medical institutions qualified for liver transplantation

By December 31st, 2023, a total of 118 medical institutions were qualified to perform liver transplantation. The top ten provinces (autonomous regions and municipalities) with the greatest number of liver transplant centers were Beijing (13), Guangdong (12), Shanghai (10), Shandong (8), Fujian (7), Zhejiang (7), Hubei (6), Guangxi (5), Hunan (5), and Chongqing (5) (Figure 4-1).

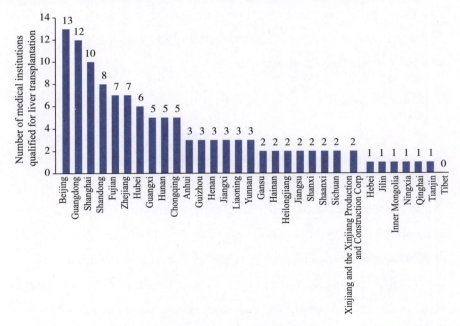

Figure 4-1 Distribution of medical institutions with liver transplant qualifications of each province (autonomous region and municipality) of China in 2023

Chapter 4 Liver Transplantation in China

From 2015 to 2023, a total of 48 515 cases of liver transplantation have been performed in China, including 41 866 cases of deceased donor liver transplantation (DDLT, 86.3%), and 6 649 cases of living related donor liver transplantation (LDLT, 13.7%) (Figure4-2). There were 39 802 adult liver transplantation (82.0%) and 8 713 pediatric liver transplantation (18.0%).

In 2023, 6 896 cases of liver transplantation were performed across the country, including 5 972 cases of DDLT (86.6%) and 924 cases of LDLT (13.4%), among which 6 cases were domino liver transplantation. There were 5 687 cases of adult liver transplantation (82.5%) and 1 209 cases of pediatric liver transplantation (17.5%). The top ten provinces (autonomous regions and municipalities) with the greatest number of liver transplantation performed in 2023 were Shanghai (1 208), Zhejiang (746), Guangdong (666), Beijing (557), Shandong (481), Hubei (345), Guangxi (336), Sichuan (261), Henan (241) and Tianjin (241). 20 provinces (autonomous regions and municipalities) performed more than 100 cases of liver transplantation in 2023; the total amount of liver transplantation performed in these provinces accounted for 94.9% of all cases in China (Figure 4-3). No liver transplantation was performed in Qinghai and Tibet.

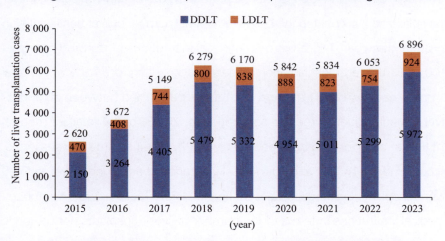

Figure 4-2 Number of liver transplantation cases from 2015 to 2023 in China

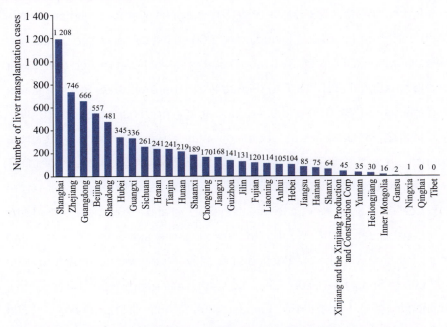

Figure 4-3 Distribution of liver transplantation cases by provinces (autonomous regions and municipalities) of China in 2023

In 2023, a total of 110 medical institutions conducted liver transplantation, among which 12 medical institutions performed more than 150 cases of liver transplantation, accounted for 42.9% of the total number of liver transplantation in China that year. There were 10 medical institutions performed between 100 and 149 liver transplantation surgeries, accounting for 17.9% of the total number nationwide; 21 medical institutions performed between 50 and 99 liver transplantation surgeries, accounting for 20.8% of the total; 27 medical institutions performed between 20 and 49 liver transplantation surgeries, accounting for 14.1%; and 40 medical institutions performed fewer than 20 liver transplantation surgeries, accounting for 4.3%. Table 4–1 lists the top ten medical institutions in terms of the number of liver transplants performed in 2023.

Chapter 4 Liver Transplantation in China

Table 4-1 Top ten medical institutions with the highest number of liver transplant cases in China in 2023

Region	Name of medical institution	Number of cases
Shanghai	Renji Hospital, Shanghai Jiao Tong University School of Medicine	583
Zhejiang	The First Affiliated Hospital, Zhejiang University School of Medicine	351
Shanghai	Huashan Hospital, Fudan University	280
Tianjin	Tianjin First Central Hospital	241
Sichuan	West China Hospital of Sichuan University	226
Shanghai	Zhongshan Hospital, Fudan University	206
Shandong	The Affiliated Hospital of Qingdao University	203
Henan	The First Affiliated Hospital of Zhengzhou University	199
Zhejiang	Shulan (Hangzhou) Hospital	175
Guangxi	The Second Affiliated Hospital of Guangxi Medical University	171

4.2 Demographic characteristics of liver transplant recipients

In 2023, the average age of liver transplant recipients in China was 43.0, with a median of 49.8. The average body mass index (BMI) of liver transplant recipients was 22.4 kg/m^2, with a median of 22.5 kg/m^2. The majority of the recipients were male (73.8%). The blood types of the recipients were mainly Type O, Type A and Type B, each accounting for around 30%. Recipients with blood type AB had the lowest proportion (Table 4-2).

Table 4-2 Demographic characteristics of liver transplant recipients in 2023

Variables	Mean ± SD	Proportion (%)	Variables	Proportion (%)
Age / Years	43.0±20.6	—	Blood Type	
BMI (kg/m^2)	22.4±4.5	—	Type O	31.0
Gender			Type A	30.7
Male	—	73.8	Type B	28.0
Female	—	26.2	Type AB	10.3

4.3 Quality and safety analysis of liver transplantation

4.3.1 The major clinical indications for liver transplantation

In 2023, the mean cold ischemia time, mean length of anhepatic phase, mean intraoperative blood loss, and mean volume of red blood cell (RBC) transfusion of LDLT in China were lower than those of DDLT. The average length of operation of LDLT was slightly higher than that of DDLT. The comparison of the mean values of importaat clinical indicators between the periods of 2015–2022 and 2023 is shown in Figures 4–4 to 4–8.

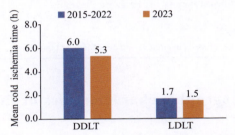

Figure 4-4　Mean cold ischemia time of liver transplantation in China

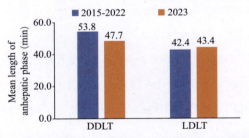

Figure 4-5　Mean length of anhepatic phase of liver transplantation in China

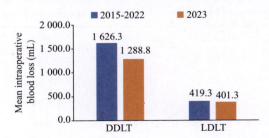

Figure 4-6　Mean intraoperative blood loss of liver transplantation in China

Chapter 4　Liver Transplantation in China

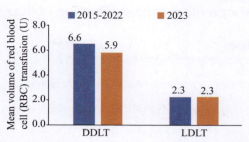

Figure 4-7　Mean volume of red blood cell (RBC) transfusion of liver transplantation in China

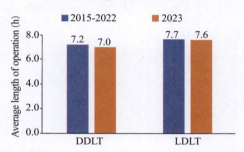

Figure 4-8　Average length of operation of liver transplantation in China

4.3.2　Pre - and post-operation variation of total serum bilirubin

The pre – and post–operation variation of total serum bilirubin in DDLT recipients and LDLT recipients in 2023 were analyzed. Results showed that the mean value of total serum bilirubin decreased significantly in post–operation recipients (Table 4–3).

Table 4-3　Mean value of the pre- and post-operation total serum bilirubin of liver transplantation in 2023

Unit: μmol/L

Time	DDLT	LDLT
pre-operation	215.5	190.9
1-week post-operation	68.0	48.3
2-week post-operation	49.0	26.8
1-month post-operation	32.5	18.1
3-month post-operation	21.1	10.5
6-month post-operation	20.8	9.7

4.3.3 Post-operation clinical situation of liver transplantation recipients

(1) 30-day post-operation complications. In 2023, the occurrence rate of 30-day post-operation complications of DDLT recipients was 24.0%. Pleural effusion (14.6%), post-operation infection (9.3%), and ascites/peritoneal abscess (8.9%) were the major complications. The occurrence rate of 30-day post-operation complications of LDLT recipients was 21.0%. Post-operation infection (13.7%), pleural effusion (10.5%), and ascites/peritoneal abscess (9.7%) were the major types.

(2) 30-day post-operation mortality rate. In 2023, the 30-day post-operation mortality rate of DDLT recipients was 4.9%, which of LDLT recipients was 2.1%.

(3) Survival rate of recipients and transplant grafts after liver transplantation. We analyzed the data from 2015 to 2023 to see the survival rate of liver transplant recipients and transplant grafts. The results are shown below.

The 1-year, 3-year, 5-year survival rate of DDLT recipients in China were 84.2%, 74.9%, and 69.3%; the 1-year, 3-year, 5-year survival rate of LDLT recipients were 93.6%, 91.8%, and 91.3%.

In terms of transplant grafts, their cumulative survival rates of DDLT in China were 83.4% at 1-year, 73.9% at 3-year, and 68.2% at 5-year; while cumulative graft survival rates of LDLT were 92.9% at 1-year, 90.8% at 3-year, and 90.0% at 5-year (Table 4-4).

(4) Tumor-free survival after liver transplantation of hepatocellular carcinoma patients. From 2015 to 2023, the 1-year, 3-year, and 5-year tumor-free survival after liver transplantation of hepatocellular carcinoma patients were 75.0%, 61.0%, and 54.1%.

Table 4-4 Survival rate of recipients and grafts after liver transplantation in China from 2015 to 2023

Unit: %

Type	1-year post-operative		3-year post-operative		5-year post-operative	
	Recipients	Grafts	Recipients	Grafts	Recipients	Grafts
DDLT	84.2	83.4	74.9	73.9	69.3	68.2
LDLT	93.6	92.9	91.8	90.8	91.3	90.0

4.4 Feature and future outlook

4.4.1 The number of liver transplants has reached a historic high

Amidst strong national policy direction, ongoing enhancements in laws and regulations, and swift progress in medical standards, the collaborative efforts of transplantation experts and scholars nationwide have led to a steady increase in the scale of liver transplantation in China, accompanied by ongoing improvements in transplant quality and technological innovation. In 2023, China ranked second worldwide in liver transplantation, with the total surpassing 6 800 cases, marking a record high for the year.

4.4.2 The recipients' age distribution is relatively concentrated, and pediatric liver transplantation is growing steadily in China

Comparing the age distribution of liver transplantation recipients in China and the United States reveals that the majority of recipients in both nations are between the ages of 50 to 64. This age group comprises 41.9% of recipients in China and 44.5% of recipients in the United States.

As China's pediatric liver transplantation technology matures, its quantity and quality have also steadily increased. Since 2018, the annual number of cases of pediatric liver transplantation performed in China has exceeded

1 000. In 2023, China performed 1 209 pediatric liver transplants, with those for children under six years old being the majority, accounting for 80.4% of all pediatric liver transplantation surgeries. In the United States, 534 pediatric liver transplantation surgeries were performed, with children under six years old accounting for 62.5% of all.

4.4.3 Actively expand source of liver donors

LDLT and split liver transplantation (SLT) are crucial methods for expanding the liver donor pool. More than 50 transplant centers have performed these kinds of liver transplantation in 2023, with significant regional variations in terms of scale. The top three provinces (autonomous regions and municipalities) with the largest numbers of LDLT were Shanghai (336), Zhejiang (169), and Tianjin (119), accounting for 67.5% of all LDLT in China. The top three provinces (autonomous regions and municipalities) with the largest numbers of SLT were Zhejiang (217), Shanghai (75), and Guangdong (58), accounting for 68.0% of all SLT in China.

4.4.4 Continuously promote refined management in liver transplantation

Under the leadership of the National Health Commission, flight inspections and research work have been conducted focusing on clinical techniques and postoperative management levels in liver transplantation, alongside data reported to the CLTR system. The National Liver Transplantation Quality Control Center and the China Organ Transplant Response System (COTRS) have collaboratively conducted a nationwide audit of medical records for super-urgent liver transplantation cases (1A). Technical exchanges, promotion, and applications have been undertaken regarding complex liver transplantations and the novel "No-touch" technique for liver transplantation in cases of liver cancer. Efforts have been executed systematically in various domains,

Chapter 4　Liver Transplantation in China

including the establishment of a quality control system, the development and dissemination of standards and guidelines, technical training for liver transplantation, monitoring and feedback of quality control information, and the ongoing enhancement of medical quality and service standards in liver transplantation.

Chapter 5　Kidney Transplantation in China

Data scope

Data showed in this chapter are mainly based on data from the Chinese Scientific Registry of Kidney Transplantation (CSRKT), spanning from January 1st, 2015, to December 31st, 2023.

Statistical methods

Descriptive statistical analysis was used to demonstrate the basic characteristics of organ transplant recipients.

Chapter highlights

(1) Since 2015, the total number of kidney transplantations this year has reached an historic high: the total number in 2023 increased by 17.7% compared to 2022 (12 712 cases), including a 13.6% increase in deceased donor (DD) kidney transplantation from 2022 (10 187 cases) and a 34.4% increase in living-related donor (LD) kidney transplantation from 2022 (2 525 cases). The number of pediatric kidney transplantations continued to rebound in 2023, basically equivalent to that in 2021. In 2023, there was a breakthrough in the number of kidney-related combined multiple organ transplantation, with a 36.5% increase compared to that of 2022. In 2023, six medical institutions performed a total of seven isolated pancreas transplantation surgeries.

Chapter 5   Kidney Transplantation in China

(2) The distribution of kidney transplantation cases continues to show regional advantages and the dominance of large transplant centers: in 2023, there were 10 provinces (autonomous regions, and municipalities) that performed 600 or more kidney transplantation surgeries, accounting for 68.2% of the total number of cases nationwide. Additionally, there were 14 medical institutions that performed more than 250 kidney transplantation surgeries, accounting for 38.2% of the total.

(3) The majority of kidney transplant recipients were male. In 2023, male recipients accounted for 69.2% of kidney transplantation.

(4) The overall survival rate after kidney transplantation was satisfactory, but there's a need to enhance the management of recipients undergoing kidney-related multi-organ combined transplantation: Data for 2023 showed that the overall survival rates at 1-year, 3-year, and 5-year after kidney transplantation were satisfactory. However, the postoperative infection rate was relatively high in pancreas-kidney transplantation, and the proportion of graft loss due to recipient death was excessively high.

5.1   Distribution of medical institutions qualified for kidney transplantation

At the end of 2023, there were 149 medical institutions qualified for kidney transplantation in China. The top ten provinces (autonomous regions and municipalities) with the greatest number of qualified institutions were Guangdong (18), Beijing (13), Hunan (10), Shandong (10), Zhejiang (9), Shanghai (8), Hubei (7), Guangxi (6), Henan (6), and Jiangsu (6) (Figure 5–1).

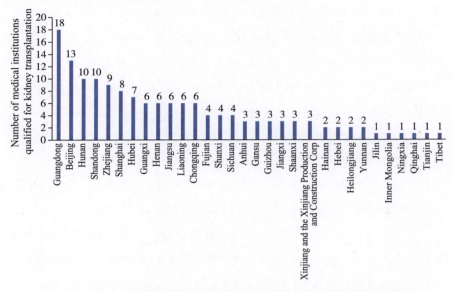

Figure 5-1 Distribution of medical institutions qualified for kidney transplantation in 2023

From 2015 to 2023, 102 761 cases of kidney transplantation had been performed in China, including 83 624 cases of DD (deceased donor) kidney transplantation and 19 137 cases of LD (living-related donor) kidney transplantation. There were 14 968 cases performed in 2023, with a 17.7% increase compared with that in 2022. Specifically, there were 11 575 cases of DD kidney transplantation, which was 13.6% higher compared with that in 2022; and 3 393 cases of LD kidney transplantation, a 34.4% increase compared with that in 2022 (Figure 5-2).

In 2023, the top ten provinces (autonomous regions and municipalities) with the most cases of kidney transplantation were Guangdong (1 626), Shandong (1 335), Hubei (1 104), Henan (1 026), Guangxi (955), Beijing (906), Sichuan (877), Zhejiang (849), Hunan (791) and Shanghai (732). The number of kidney transplant cases implemented by each province (autonomous regions and municipalities) is shown in Figure 5-3.

Chapter 5　Kidney Transplantation in China

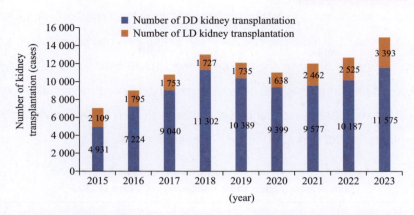

Figure 5-2　Number of kidney transplantation cases in China from 2015 to 2023

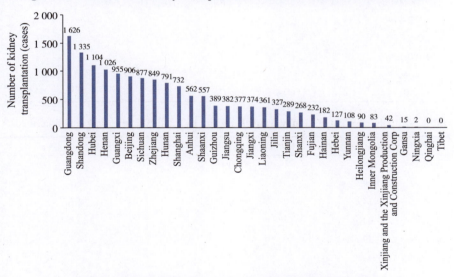

Figure 5-3　Distributions of kidney transplantation cases by province (autonomous region and municipality) of China in 2023

Regional imbalance can be seen regarding kidney transplantation in 2023. 10 provinces (autonomous regions and municipalities) have performed more than 600 cases of kidney transplantation, accounting for 68.2% of all cases (Table 5-1).

There were 14 medical institutions performed more than 250 cases of kidney transplantation, accounting for 38.2% of all cases in 2023. six

159

medical institutions had performed 200–249 cases; 35 medical institutions had performed 100–199 cases; 27 medical institutions had performed 50-99 cases; 39 medical institutions had performed 10-49 cases; and 13 medical institutions had performed 1-9 cases. Additionally, 15 medical institutions had not performed kidney transplantation, 12 of which had not performed kidney transplantation for more than three consecutive years (Table 5–2).

Table 5-1 Distribution of kidney transplantation by province (autonomous region and municipality) of China in 2023

Number of cases	Number of provinces (autonomous regions and municipalities)	Proportion (%)
≥ 600	10	68.2
400-599	2	7.5
200-399	9	20
100-199	3	2.8
1-99	5	1.5
0	2	0

Table 5-2 Distribution of kidney transplantation by medical institution of China in 2023

Number of cases	Number of medical institutions	Proportion (%)
≥ 250	14	38.2
200-249	6	9.0
100-199	35	31.6
50-99	27	13.0
10-49	39	7.7
1-9	13	0.4
0	15	0

In 2023, the top ten provinces (autonomous regions and municipalities) with the greatest number of DD kidney transplantation were Guangdong, Shandong, Guangxi, Hubei, Beijing, Henan, Hunan, Shanghai, Zhejiang and Shaanxi, accounting for 69.3% of the total number of DD cases in China (Figure 5–4). The top ten medical institutions to perform DD kidney transplantation are seen in Table 5–3.

Chapter 5 Kidney Transplantation in China

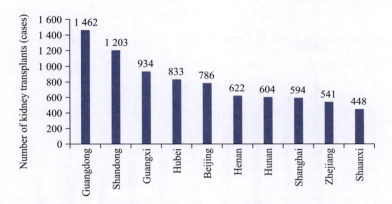

Figure 5-4 Top ten provinces (autonomous regions and municipalities) of China with the most DD kidney transplant cases in 2023

Table 5-3 Top ten medical institutions with the most cases of DD kidney transplantation across China in 2023

Region	Name of medical institutions	Number of DD cases	Number of total cases
Guangxi	The Second Affiliated Hospital of Guangxi Medical University	416	419
Shaanxi	The First Affiliated Hospital of Xi'an Jiaotong University	403	504
Henan	The First Affiliated Hospital of Zhengzhou University	368	569
Shanghai	Renji Hospital, Shanghai Jiao Tong University School of Medicine	362	439
Sichuan	West China Hospital of Sichuan University	314	711
Guangdong	The First Affiliated Hospital, Sun Yat-sen University	305	348
Zhejiang	The First Affiliated Hospital, Zhejiang University School of Medicine	295	560
Shandong	The Affiliated Hospital of Qingdao University	257	267
Hubei	Tongji Hospital Affiliated to Tongji Medical College of Huazhong University of Science &Technology	253	418
Shandong	Shandong Provincial Qianfoshan Hospital	252	276

In 2023, the top ten provinces (autonomous regions and municipalities) with the greatest number of LD kidney transplantation were Sichuan, Henan, Anhui, Zhejiang, Hubei, Tianjin, Hunan, Guangdong, Shanghai and

Shandong (Figure 5–5). The top ten medical institutions to perform LD kidney transplantation are seen in Table 5–4.

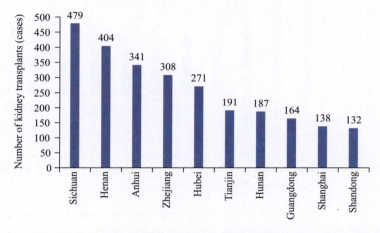

Figure 5-5　Top ten provinces (autonomous regions and municipalities) with the most living-related kidney transplantation across China in 2023

Table 5-4　Top ten medical institutions with the most LD kidney transplantation across China in 2023

Region	Name of medical institutions	Number of LD cases	Number of total cases
Sichuan	West China Hospital of Sichuan University	397	711
Zhejiang	The First Affiliated Hospital, Zhejiang University School of Medicine	265	560
Anhui	The First Affiliated Hospital of USTC	236	325
Henan	The First Affiliated Hospital of Zhengzhou University	201	569
Tianjin	Tianjin First Central Hospital	191	289
Hubei	Tongji Hospital Affiliated to Tongji Medical College of Huazhong University of Science &Technology	165	418
Hunan	The Second Xiangya Hospital of Central South University	132	267
Henan	Henan Provincial People's Hospital	118	159
Shaanxi	The First Affiliated Hospital of Xi'an Jiaotong University	101	504
Anhui	The First Affiliated Hospital of Anhui Medical University	100	194

Chapter 5 Kidney Transplantation in China

In 2023, the number of pediatric kidney transplantation (age of recipients was under 18) was 669, accounting for 4.5% of the total domestic cases of kidney transplantation in China, which was a 16.3% decrease compared to 2022 (Figure 5-6). Among these, there were 2 recipients aged under 1 year, 46 recipients aged 1 to under 6 years, 283 recipients aged 6 to under 14 years, and 338 recipients aged 14 to under 18 years.

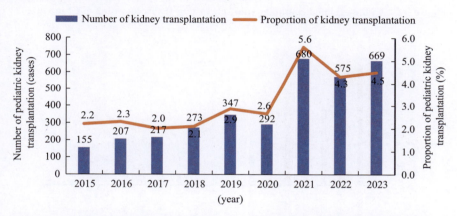

Figure 5-6 Numbers and proportions of pediatric kidney transplantation in China from 2015 to 2023

In 2023, China performed a total of 7 isolated pancreas transplantations, 1 combined liver–pancreas transplantation, and 116 kidney–related multi–organ combined transplantations, representing a 36.5% increase compared to 2022 (85 cases). Among the multi–organ transplantations, there were 42 combined liver–kidney transplantations, 68 combined pancreas–kidney transplantations, and 6 combined heart–kidney transplantations (Figure 5–7). The number of kidney–related multi–organ combined transplantations performed by each province (autonomous region, and municipality) in 2023 is shown in Figure 5–8. The medical institutions that performed isolated pancreas transplants in 2023 are listed in Table 5–5, and those that performed kidney–related multi–organ combined transplants are listed in Table 5–6.

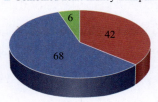

Figure 5-7 Kidney-related combined multiple organs transplantation of China in 2023

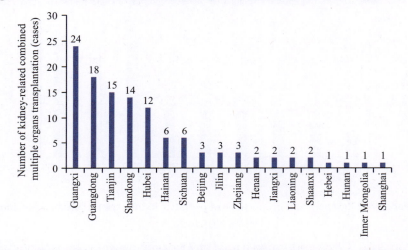

Figure 5-8 Number of kidney-related combined multiple organs transplantation in each province (autonomous region and municipality) of China in 2023

Table 5-5 Medical institutions that performed isolated pancreas transplantations in China in 2023

Region	Name of medical institution	Number of cases
Sichuan	Sichuan Provincial People's Hospital	2
Shanxi	Shanxi Bethune Hospital	1
Shandong	Shandong Provincial Qianfoshan Hospital	1
Shandong	The Affiliated Hospital of Qingdao University	1
Liaoning	The First Affiliated Hospital of USTC	1
Hubei	Tongji Hospital Affiliated to Tongji Medical College of Huazhong University of Science &Technology	1

Chapter 5　Kidney Transplantation in China

Table 5-6　Top ten medical institutions with the most cases of kidney-related combined multiple organs transplantation in China in 2023

Region	Name of medical institution	Number of cases
Guangxi	The Second Affiliated Hospital of Guangxi Medical University	21
Tianjin	Tianjin First Central Hospital	15
Hubei	Tongji Hospital Affiliated to Tongji Medical College of Huazhong University of Science &Technology	12
Guangdong	The First Affiliated Hospital, Sun Yat-sen University	9
Shandong	The Affiliated Hospital of Qingdao University	8
Hainan	The Second Affiliated Hospital of Hainan Medical University	5
Shandong	Shandong Provincial Qianfoshan Hospital	5
Guangdong	The Second Affiliated Hospital of Guangzhou Medical University	4
Sichuan	Sichuan Provincial People's Hospital	4
Jilin	Jilin University First Hospital	3

5.2　Demographic characteristics of kidney transplant recipients

In 2023, the mean age of kidney transplant recipients in China was (40.2 ± 12.5) years. with a BMI of (22.1 ± 3.6) kg/m^2 and a median pretransplant dialysis time of 662 days. The majority of the recipients were male (69.2%). The most common blood type among the recipients was Type O, accounting for 33.3%, while the least common was Type AB, accounting for 9.8% (Table 5–7).

Table 5-7　Demographic characteristics of kidney transplant recipients in China in 2023

Variables	Mean ± SD
Recipient age /years	40.2±12.5
BMI (kg/m²)	22.1±3.6
Dialysis duration	Median [IQR]
Preoperative dialysis duration/d	662（304-1 248）

	Continued
Recipient blood type	Number of cases (Proportion/%)
Type O	4 977 (33.3)
Type A	4 395 (29.4)
Type B	4 123 (27.5)
Type AB	1 473 (9.8)
Gender	Number of cases (Proportion/%)
Male	10 362 (69.2)
Female	4 606 (30.8)

Among all recipients, 677 cases were pediatric kidney transplant recipients (under 18 years) (4.5%); 2 139 recipients were aged 18 to under 30 years (14.3%); recipients aged 30 to under 50 years accounted for 8 349 cases (55.8%); 3 545 cases were recipients aged 50 to under 65 years (23.7%); transplantation among the elderly (65 years or above) accounted for 266 cases (1.8%).

5.3 Quality and safety analysis of kidney transplantation

5.3.1 Ischemia time of donor kidney

An analysis of LD (living–related donor) and DD (deceased donor) kidney transplant cases in 2023 found that the mean cold ischemia time and warm ischemia time for the donor kidneys were within the standard range (Table 5–8).

Table 5-8 Ischemia time of LD and DD kidney transplantation in 2023

Variables	LD (Mean ± SD)	DD (Mean ± SD)
Cold ischemia time of donor kidney (h)	2.1±1.6	5.8±3.9
Warm ischemia time of donor kidney (min)	3.0±2.0	5.1±3.7

In 2023, the proportion of donor kidney cold ischemia time equals to 24 hours or less in LD kidney transplantation and DD kidney transplantation was

99.7% and 98.9%, respectively; the proportion of warm ischemia time equals to 10 minutes or less was 98.6% and 72.7%. 98.6% of DD and 72.7% of LD kidney transplantation had a warm ischemia of less than 10 minutes. In 2023, 27.3% of recipients of DD kidney transplantation had a warm ischemia time of more than 10 minutes (Table 5-9).

Table 5-9 Proportion of ischemia time of LD and DD kidney transplantation in 2023

Variables	LD (%)	DD (%)
Donor kidney with cold ischemia time ≤ 24 h	99.7	98.9
Donor kidney with warm ischemia time ≤ 10 min	98.6	72.7

5.3.2 Changes of serum creatinine value in the pre-and post-kidney transplant recipients

An analysis of serum creatinine value at four time points—pre-operation, 30-day post-operation, 180-day post-operation, and 360-day post-operation—for kidney transplantation cases in 2023 revealed the mean serum creatinine value for LD and DD kidney transplantation recipients as shown in Table 5-10. An analysis of cases from 2015 to 2023 showed that the average serum creatinine value at preoperative and various postoperative time points for LD and DD kidney transplants were as follows: 996.5 μmol/L and 941.3 μmol/L at pre-operation; 125.7 μmol/L and 151.6 μmol/L at 30-day post-operation, 120.6 μmol/L and 128.6 μmol/L at 180-day post-operation, and 97.3 μmol/L and 118.2 μmol/L at 360-day post-operation, respectively.

Table 5-10 Mean values of serum creatinine in the pre- and post-operation kidney transplant recipients in 2023

Time point	LD (μmol/L)	DD (μmol/L)
Pre-operation	996.5	941.3
30-day post-operation	125.7	151.6
180-day post-operation	120.6	128.6
360-day post-operation	97.3	118.2

5.3.3 Overview of adverse events in post-operation period of kidney transplantation

In general, the adverse events in post–operation period mainly include delayed renal graft function, acute rejection, infections, all–cause graft loss and recipient death. An analysis of the follow–up data for cases in 2023 revealed the incidence rates of major adverse events as shown in Table 5–11. The 30–day post–operation mortality rate was 0.3%. In the meantime, Table 5–12 showed the rate of major adverse events following combined multiple organs transplantation related to kidney.

Table 5-11 Rates of post-operation adverse event of kidney transplantation in China in 2023

Adverse events	LD (%)	DD (%)
Delayed renal graft function	1.9	14.9
Acute rejection	1.7	3.3
Infections	4.0	7.7
All-cause graft loss	1.6	4.4
Recipient death	0.2	1.2

Table 5-12 Rates of post-operation adverse event of kidney-related combined multiple organs transplantation in China in 2023

Adverse events	Incidence rate (%)
Delayed renal graft function	7.8
Acute rejection	2.6
Infections	9.6
All-cause graft loss	10.4
Recipient death	6.1

5.3.4 Survival analysis of kidney transplant recipients and grafts

A survival analysis was conducted on 102 761 kidney transplant recipients/grafts (hereinafter referred to as "patient/kidney") performed in China between 2015 and 2023. The Kaplan–Meier method was utilized to calculate cumulative survival rates. The 1-year post-operation patient/kidney survival rates for LD kidney transplantation were 99.1%/98.4%, and for DD kidney transplants were 97.5%/95.5%; the 3-year patient/kidney survival rates for LD kidney transplantation were 98.5%/96.3%, and for DD kidney transplantation were 96.2%/92.6%; the 5-year patient/kidney survival rates for LD kidney transplantation were 97.8%/93.1%, and for DD kidney transplantation were 94.7%/88.8% (table 5-13).

Table 5-13 Postoperative survival rates for kidney transplantation recipients/kidney grafts in China, from 2015 to 2023

Unit: %

Donor types	1-year post-operation		3-year post-operation		5-year post-operation	
	Recipients	Grafts	Recipients	Grafts	Recipients	Grafts
LD kidney	99.1	98.4	98.5	96.3	97.8	93.1
DD kidney	97.5	95.5	96.2	92.6	94.7	88.8

5.4 Feature and future outlook

5.4.1 The total number of kidney transplants reached a historic high, with a notable increase in the number of LD kidney transplants

In 2023, the number of kidney transplantation in China attained a record high, exhibiting a 17.7% increase in total cases compared to 2022 (12 712 cases). There was a substantial rise in living donor kidney transplantation, totaling 3 393 cases, marking the highest figure on record and a 34.4% increase relative to 2022. The significant increase in transplantation numbers not only indicates the advanced system and management framework for deceased donor organ donation in China but also implies the positive outcomes linked to living donor kidney transplantation. This may be attributed to the optimization of living organ donation processes and enhanced operational efficiency at numerous transplant centers.

5.4.2 The number of pediatric kidney transplants has rebounded

The number of pediatric kidney transplants has been continuously rising in recent years. In 2023, the total number of cases reached 669, reflecting a 16.3% increase from 2022, comprising 45 cases (6.7%) of living–donor kidney transplantation and 624 cases (93.3%) of deceased–donor kidney transplantation. Regarding age distribution, 331 recipients (48.4%) were 14 years of age or younger. Of the recipients, 589 (88.0%) received kidney donated by children, including 37 cases (5.5%) where the donor was under 1 year old. This indicates that kidney transplantation utilizing kidneys from younger or lower–weight children is progressively being implemented in clinical practice. The efficient and effective utilization of kidneys donated by younger or lower–weight children in organ donation and transplantation surgery management is a significant topic for discussion.

5.4.3 The distribution of kidney transplant cases continues to show regional and large transplant center advantages

In 2023, the ten provinces (autonomous regions and municipalities) with the highest number of kidney transplantation cases were Guangdong, Shandong, Hubei, Henan, Guangxi, Beijing, Sichuan, Zhejiang, Hunan, and Shanghai, collectively representing 68.2% of the national total, indicating a distinct regional predominance. In 2023, 14 medical institutions conducted 250 or more kidney transplants, an increase of four from 2022, representing 38.2% of the nation's total kidney transplant cases. 55 medical institutions conducted 100 or more kidney transplants, representing 78.8% of the national total. Furthermore, a medical institution exceeded 700 cases, underscoring the substantial case volume advantage of large transplant centers.

5.4.4 Attention should be paid to multi-organ combined transplantation

In 2023, the number of kidney-related multi-organ combined transplantation cases rose by 36.5% compared to 2022. Seven medical institutions conducted seven isolated pancreas transplantation surgeries. In comparison to isolated kidney transplantation, simultaneous pancreas-kidney transplantation exhibits a comparatively elevated incidence of postoperative complications, notably all-cause graft loss and recipient mortality.

5.4.5 Emphasis should be placed on research hotspots in kidney transplantation and the revision of clinical guidelines

To further promote homogeneous management in clinical diagnosis and treatment of kidney transplantation and improve the quality of medical services for kidney transplantation, multiple clinical guidelines are currently being developed or revised. Furthermore, experts and scholars in China are investigating and developing consensus and guidelines tailored to the nation's specific circumstances, focusing on emerging issues in kidney donation and transplantation, including the rational allocation and use of kidneys donated by younger or lower-weight children, as well as the scientific management of pancreas transplantation and simultaneous pancreas-kidney transplantation.

Chapter 6 Heart Transplantation in China

Data scope

Data showed in this chapter are mainly based on data from the China Heart Transplant Registry (CHTR), spanning from January 1st, 2015, to December 31st, 2023.

Statistical methods

Descriptive statistical analysis was used to demonstrate the basic situation of heart transplantation surgeries, and survival analysis methods were employed to calculate the cumulative survival rate.

Chapter highlights

(1) In recent years, the number of heart transplantation in China has increased year by year, reaching 994 cases in 2023, an increase of 40% compared to 2022. There are a total of 76 hospitals qualified for heart transplantation nationwide, distributed across 29 provinces, indicating that medical accessibility has been expanding annually.

(2) Quality indicators such as the pre-heart transplantation cardiopulmonary exercise testing rate, donor heart ischemia time, and post-operative in-hospital outcomes have continued to improve.

(3) The survival rates at 30-day, 1-year, 3-year, and 5-year after heart transplantation were 93.1%, 81.5%, 76.1%, and 70.2% respectively, reaching

Chapter 6 Heart Transplantation in China

international standards.

6.1 Distribution of medical institutions qualified for heart transplantation

At the end of 2023, a total of 76 medical institutions in China were qualified for heart transplantation. Provinces (autonomous regions and municipalities) with the largest number of heart transplant hospitals are Guangdong (8), Zhejiang (7), Beijing (5), Shanghai (5), and Hubei (5) (Figure 6-1).

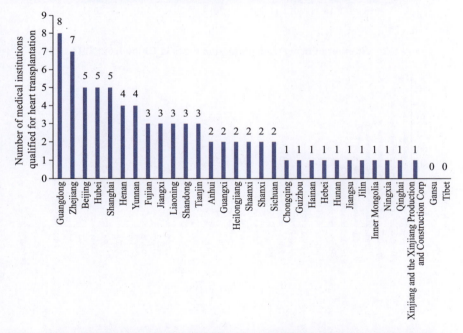

Figure 6-1 Distribution of medical institutions qualified for heart transplantation in provinces (autonomous regions and municipalities) of China in 2023

From 2015 to 2023, a total of 5 261 heart transplantation were reported in China (Figure 6-2). In 2023, 994 cases of heart transplantation were performed in China, an 40% increase compared to 2022, including 125 cases of pediatric (age under 18) heart transplantation accounting for 12.6% of the total, and two cases of heart-lung combined transplantation. Distribution of cases of heart transplantation of each province (autonomous region and municipality) is shown in Figure 6-3.

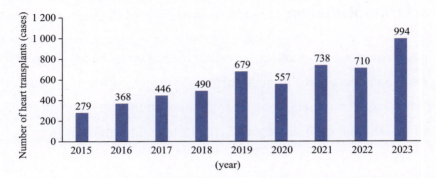

Figure 6-2   Number of heart transplantation cases in China from 2015 to 2023

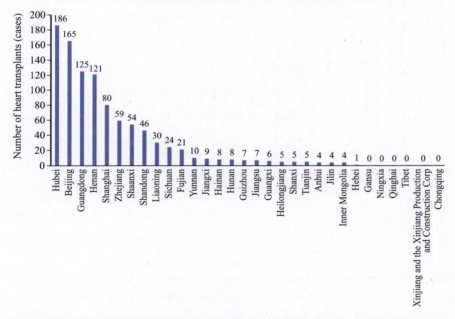

Figure 6-3   Distribution of heart transplant cases in each province (autonomous region and municipality) of China in 2023

In 2023, a total of 64 medical institutions nationwide conducted heart transplantation surgeries. Among them, 2 medical institutions performed more than 100 cases, and two medical institutions performed more than 50 cases (Figure 6–4). The top ten medical institutions in China in terms of the number of heart transplantation cases in 2023 are shown in Figure 6–5.

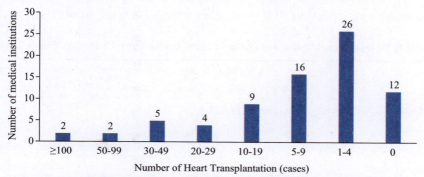

Figure 6-4 Distribution of heart transplantation cases by Chinese medical institutions in 2023

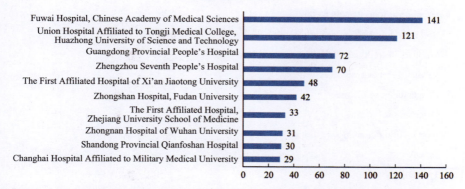

Figure 6-5 Top ten medical institations with the highest number of heart transplantation cases in China in 2023

6.2 Demographic characteristics of heart transplant recipients

In 2023, the median age of heart transplantation recipients was 50.0 years old. The majority of the recipients were male (76.7%). The median BMI of recipients was 22.2 kg/m^2. As for the blood types of transplant recipients, Type O accounted for 28.0%, Type A accounted for 33.0%, Type B accounted for 29.2%, and Type AB accounted for 9.9%. The median age of adult transplant recipients was 53.0 years, of which 78.8% were males. The median age of pediatric transplant recipients was 11.0 years, of which 63.2% were males (Table 6-1).

Table 6-1 Demographic characteristics of heart transplant recipients in China in 2023

Variables	Total (n=994)	Adult recipients (n=869)	Pediatric recipients (n=125)
Median age, IQR (years)	50.0 (34.0,58.0)	53.0 (42.0,59.0)	11.0 (7.0, 14.0)
Male/%	76.7	78.8	63.2
Median weight, IQR (kg)	64.0 (51.7,71.6)	65.0 (56.0,73.0)	33.7 (21.0,47.5)
Median height, IQR (cm)	168.5 (160.0, 173.0)	170.0 (163.0, 174.0)	145.0 (127.0, 165.0)
Median BMI, IQR (kg/m^2)	22.2 (19.1, 24.7)	22.6 (20.2, 25.1)	15.6 (13.2, 19.7)
Cause of heart transplantation (%)			
Non-ischemic cardiomyopathy	76.8	75.8	83.5
Coronary heart disease	12.6	14.4	0.8
Valvular heart disease	3.1	3.4	1.5
Congenital heart disease	2.2	1.3	8.3
Other causes	5.3	5.1	5.9
Proportion of different blood types (%)			
Type A	33.0	33.5	28.6
Type B	29.2	30.1	22.4
Type O	28.0	26.1	40.8
Type AB	9.9	10.3	7.2

The main causes of recipients demanding heart transplantation were non-ischemic cardiomyopathy and coronary heart disease, accounting for 76.8% and 12.6%, respectively, followed by valvular heart disease (3.1%), and congenital heart disease (2.2%). The main causes of adult recipients were non-ischemic cardiomyopathy (75.8%), and coronary heart disease (14.4%); the main causes of pediatric recipients are non-ischemic cardiomyopathy (83.5%), and congenital heart disease (8.3%).

6.3 Quality and safety analysis of heart transplantation

6.3.1 Rate of pre-operation cardiopulmonary exercise test

Cardiopulmonary exercise test is the preferred method to determine whether a patient meets the criteria for heart transplantation. For transplant candidates without contraindications for cardiopulmonary exercise test, using this test for heart transplant assessment can help doctors understand whether the functional status of organs other than the heart of the transplant recipient is normal and to promptly address any existing issues.

In 2023, rate of pre-operation cardiopulmonary exercise test for adult heart transplant recipients were 57.2%, a 12.8% improvement than that of 2022 (Table 6-2).

Table 6-2 Rate of pre-operation cardiopulmonary exercise test in China in 2022 and 2023

Year	Rate of pre-operation cardiopulmonary exercise test (%)
2022	44.4
2023	57.2

6.3.2 Ischemia time of donor heart

The ischemic time of the donor heart refers to the period from the time the donor heart is procured until it is implanted into the recipient. Studies have shown that donor heart preservation techniques generally allow for a safe ischemic time of 6 hours or less. The proportion of donor hearts with an ischemic time of 6 hours or less is an important indicator reflecting the standardization of donor heart selection and maintenance practices at medical institutions.

In 2023, the median ischemic time of donor hearts for heart transplantation was 3.3 hours, a decrease of 0.3 hours compared to the median ischemic time in 2022 (Table 6-3). The proportion of transplant patients with a donor heart ischemic time of 6 hours or less was 85.3%.

Table 6-3 Ischemia time of heart transplantation in China in 2022 and 2023

Year	Donor heart Ischemia time, IQR/(h)	Proportion of ischemia time ≤ 6 hours (%)
2022	3.6（2.5, 5.5）	88.0
2023	3.3（2.3, 5.3）	85.3

6.3.3 Post-operation in-hospital survival

In 2023, the in-hospital survival rate of heart transplant recipients in China was 94.2%. The incidence rate of post-operation infections among heart transplant recipients was 16.7%, other major post-operation complications were cardiac arrest (3.8%), reoperation (4.6%), tracheotomy (5.1%), and reintubation (9.6%). Multiple organ failure, allograft heart failure, and infection all accounted for 11.3%, 6.5%, and 32.3%, respectively in the causes of the in-hospital deaths of heart transplant recipients (Table 6-4).

Table 6-4 In-hospital post-operation survival of heart transplant recipients in 2023

Variable	Proportion (%)		
	Total (n=994)	Adult recipients (n=869)	Pediatric recipients (n=125)
In-hospital survival	94.2	93.6	97.7
Post-operation complications			
Infection	16.7	16.9	9.8
Cardiac arrest	3.8	6.8	8.3
Reoperation	4.6	6.5	9.8
Tracheotomy	5.1	6.7	9.8
Reintubation	9.6	6.5	8.3
Cause of in-hospital death			
Multiple organ failure	11.3	11.9	0
Allograft heart failure	6.5	6.8	0
Infection	32.3	33.9	0
Cerebrovascular causes	27.4	23.7	100
Acute rejection	6.5	6.8	0
Others	16	16.9	0

6.3.4 Survival analysis

From 2015 to 2023, the survival rate of 30-day, 1-year, and 3-year and 5-year post-operation of heart transplantation in China were 93.1%, 81.5%, 76.1% and 70.2%, respectively. The corresponding survival rates among adult recipients were 92.2%, 80.8%, 75.6% and 70.6%, respectively. The corresponding survival rates among pediatric recipients were 94.8%, 87.2%, 81.6% and 73.3%, respectively (Table 6-5).

Table 6-5 Survival rate post-operation of heart transplantation from 2015 to 2023

Unit: %

	Post-operation 30-day survival rate	Post-operation 1-year survival rate	Post-operation 3-year survival rate	Post-operation 5-year survival rate
Total	93.1	81.5	76.1	70.2
Adult recipients	92.2	80.8	75.6	70.6
Pediatric recipients	94.8	87.2	81.6	73.3

6.4 Feature and future outlook

6.4.1 The number of heart transplantation has increased year by year, with significant differences among medical institutions

In recent years, heart transplantation in China has developed rapidly, with the number of heart transplants increasing annually. In 2023, a total of 994 heart transplants were performed, representing a 40% increase compared to 2022. Except for Tibet and Gansu, all provinces (autonomous regions and municipalities) have medical institutions capable of performing heart transplants, providing high accessibility to heart transplant medical services for patients.

Fuwai Hospital, Chinese Academy of Medical Sciences, and Union

Hospital, Tongji Medical College, Huazhong University of Science and Technology, each conduct over 100 heart transplants annually, achieving world-leading levels in both transplant volume and quality. Medical institutions such as Guangdong Provincial People's Hospital, Zhongshan Hospital Fudan University, and Zhengzhou Seventh People's Hospital maintain an average of around 50 heart transplantations annually, demonstrating relatively stable heart transplantation service capabilities. Nonetheless, substantial disparities in technical capabilities persist among medical institutions. In 2023, 12 medical institutions nationwide did not conduct any heart transplants, while 42 institutions performed fewer than ten heart transplants. These medical institutions are qualified for heart transplants but have not successfully delivered or executed clinical heart transplant services.

Consequently, the subsequent emphasis on enhancing the quality of heart transplantation across the nation will involve the establishment of a peer-to-peer support framework among medical institutions, alongside the promotion of the heart transplant management expertise and developmental principles of exemplary medical institutions.

6.4.2 The shortage of heart donors remains a significant constraint on the growth of heart transplantations cases

Currently, the growth in the number of heart transplantation in China remains constrained by the shortage of donor organs. Data from the China Organ Transplant Response System (COTRS) indicates that in 2023, the heart recovery rate per donor in China was 0.16, which is inferior to that of developed nations. Between 2020 and 2023, the percentage of organ donors of brain death considerably rose, attaining 70.7% in 2023, thereby presenting substantial potential for enhancing the heart donation rate.

In 2024, the National Heart Transplantation Quality Control Center will collaborate with the OPQC and the Big Data Center of National Health Commission for Human Tissue and Organ Transplant and Medicine to provide nationwide training for donor hospitals with heart donors. The objective is to enhance the competencies of OPOs and transplant hospitals in donor evaluation, preservation, and procurement, consequently elevating the donation rate and the quality of donated hearts.

6.4.3 Further enhance the training and team building of heart transplant surgeons

The rapid development of heart transplantation in China has been significantly attributed to the robust support from transplant surgeon teams across diverse medical institutions. Nonetheless, the existing quantity of heart transplant surgeons in China remains insufficient to satisfy the rising demand. In 2023, the average number of heart transplant surgeons in authorized medical institutions was 3.1, of which only 85 surgeons conducted heart transplant surgeries. The training and certification of heart transplant internists require attention as well. Currently, the qualification certification standards for heart transplant physicians in China are limited to surgeons, despite the fact that the diagnostic and therapeutic processes of heart transplantation, encompassing pre-transplant evaluation, postoperative rehabilitation, and long-term follow-up, necessitate substantial involvement from internists.

Therefore, further emphasis needs to be placed on the technical skill training of heart transplant internists and surgeons, as well as the training of transplant teams. Relevant training standards and systems should be established. Meanwhile, medical institution teams that have not performed heart transplants should receive retraining.

6.4.4 Continuously advance quality improvement initiatives for heart transplantations

Since 2021, the National Heart Transplantation Quality Control Center has been committed to enhancing the transplant quality of medical institutions nationwide by issuing technical specifications and providing pertinent training. A notable quality improvement initiative is the augmentation of preoperative cardiopulmonary exercise testing (CPET) rates, which rose from 44.4% in 2022 to 57.2% in 2023, thereby consistently refined preoperative evaluation and recipient selection for heart transplantation.

In 2024, the National Heart Transplantation Quality Control Center will persist in enhancing quality improvement initiatives centered on vital aspects of heart transplantation. Efforts will be concentrated on performing quality reviews and enhancing the management of postoperative complications and follow-up care after heart transplantation. The Center will formulate clinical guidelines for heart transplantation in China, thereby advancing the standardization of clinical diagnosis and treatment in this field.

Chapter 7　Lung Transplantation in China

Data scope

Data showed in this chapter are mainly based on data from the China Lung Transplantation Registry (CLuTR), spanning from January 1st, 2015, to December 31st, 2023.

Statistical methods

Descriptive statistical analysis was used to describe the basic situation of lung transplantation in China, and Kaplan-Meier method was employed to calculate the cumulative survival rate.

Chapter highlights

(1) In 2023, a total of 959 lung transplantation surgeries were performed in China, including 361 single lung transplantations (37.6%), 596 double lung transplantations (62.2%), and two heart-lung combined transplantations (0.2%). Among the adult lung transplant recipients in China, males accounted for 85.1%, with an average age of (42.3 ± 12.8) years. The top six medical institutions accounted for 69.5% of the total number of lung transplantations. Therefore, measures should be taken to further promote the balanced development of lung transplantation among medical institutions.

(2) In 2023, the survival rate of 30-day post-operation of lung transplant recipients reached 83.8%. The incidence rates of tracheal anastomotic lesions

and acute rejection after transplantation declined, but the incidence rates of primary graft dysfunction and perioperative infections increased. Therefore, it is necessary to further strengthen the monitoring and dynamic feedback of quality control indicators, and continuously promote a comprehensive and multi-faceted mechanism for the prevention and control of complications throughout the process.

(3) In 2023, China completed 22 pediatric lung transplants, with 14 cases performed by the Second Affiliated Hospital, Zhejiang University School of Medicine, and six cases by Wuxi People's Hospital. Male recipients accounted for 63.6% of pediatric lung transplants in China, with an average age of (12.5 ± 3.5) years. The 30-day survival rate after surgery exceeded 90%, suggesting that pediatric lung transplant technology is gradually improving and maturing. In order to promote substantial development of this technology and improve long-term prognosis, it is urgently needed to develop technical guidance for pediatric lung transplantation based on China's conditions.

7.1 Distribution of medical institutions qualified for lung transplantation

As of the end of 2023, a total of 60 medical institutions in China have obtained lung transplant qualifications, covering 24 provinces (autonomous regions and municipalities). The number of medical institutions qualified for lung transplantation in each province (autonomous region and municipality) of China is shown in Figure 7–1.

From 2015 to 2023, 4 558 cases of lung transplantation have been reported through CLuTR. Over the years, 118, 204, 299, 403, 489, 513, 775, 798 and 959 cases have been performed each year (Figure 7–2), showing an upward trend over time. Among them, a total of 69 pediatric lung transplantation surgeries were reported, with the number of surgeries conducted annually being 2, 1, 0, 3, 9, 8, 12, 12, and 22, respectively (Figure 7-3).

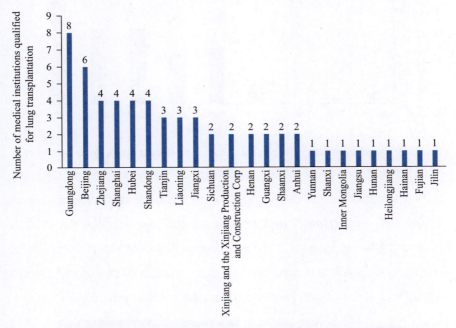

Figure7-1　Distribution of medical institutions qualified for lung transplantation of each province (autonomous region and municipality) of China in 2023

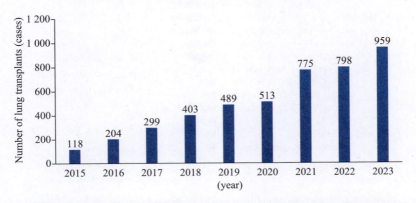

Figure 7-2　Number of lung transplantation cases in China from 2015 to 2023

Report on Organ Donation and Transplantation in China (2023)

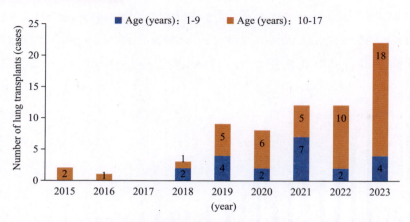

Figure 7-3 Number of pediatric lung transplantation cases in China from 2015 to 2023

In 2023, 43 medical institutions performed lung transplantation surgeries. The medical institutions that performed 10 or more lung transplantations are shown in Figure 7–4. Among the 22 pediatric lung transplantations performed in 2023, the Second Affiliated Hospital Zhejiang University School of Medicine completed 14 cases, Wuxi People's Hospital completed six cases, and Chinese PLA General Hospital and China–Japan Friendship Hospital each completed one case.

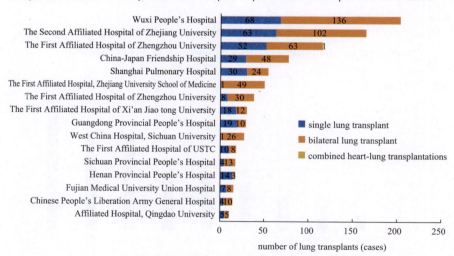

Figure 7-4 Ranking of medical institutions performing ten or more lung transplantations in 2023

7.2 Demographic characteristics of lung transplant recipients

In 2023, among adult lung transplant recipients in China, males accounted for 85.1%, with a mean age of (42.3 ± 12.8) years, and 47.8% were over 60 years old. Blood Types O, A, B, and AB accounted for 33.5%, 29.1%, 26.7% and 10.7%, respectively. Before transplantation, 15.9% of the recipients were hospitalized in the ICU. In terms of cardiac function, the proportions of recipients with complete limitation of daily activities (NYHA Class IV) and those in severe condition requiring hospitalization were 20.3% and 21.6%, respectively. For pediatric lung transplant recipients in China in 2023, males accounted for 63.6%, with a mean age of 12.5 ± 3.5 years. Blood Types O, A, B, and AB accounted for 50.0%, 36.4%, 9.1% and 4.5%, respectively. Before transplantation, 13.6% of the pediatric recipients were hospitalized in the ICU. In terms of cardiac function, the proportions of recipients with complete limitation of daily activities (NYHA Class IV) and those in severe condition requiring hospitalization were 13.6% and 27.3%, respectively (Table 7–1).

Table 7-1 Demographic characteristics of lung transplant recipients in 2023

Variables (Adult recipients)	Proportion (%)	Variables (Pediatric recipients)	Proportion (%)
Gender		Gender	
Male	85.1	Male	63.6
Female	14.9	Female	36.4
Age(year)		Age (year)	
18-35	7.0	1-9	18.2
36-49	14.0	10-17	81.8
50-59	31.2		–
60-64	16.5		–
65-74	29.8		–
≥ 75	1.5		–

			Continued
Variables (Adult recipients)	Proportion (%)	Variables (Pediatric recipients)	Proportion (%)
Blood Type		Blood Type	
Type O	33.5	Type O	50.0
Type A	29.1	Type A	36.4
Type B	26.7	Type B	9.1
Type AB	10.7	Type AB	4.5
Hospitalization before transplantation		Hospitalization before transplantation	
ICU	15.9	ICU	13.6
Regular hospitalization	69.7	Regular hospitalization	77.3
Not hospitalized	14.4	Not hospitalized	9.1
Pre-transplantation heart function		Pre-transplantation heart function	
No activity restrictions (NYHA I/II)	1.4	No activity restrictions (NYHA I/II)	0.0
Partially limited daily activities (NYHA III)	56.7	Partially limited daily activities (NYHA III)	59.1
Completely restricted daily activities (NYHA IV)	20.3	Completely restricted daily activities (NYHA IV)	13.6
Serious illness requiring hospitalization	21.6	Serious illness requiring hospitalization	27.3

In 2023, the primary diseases of adult lung transplant recipients in China were mainly idiopathic pulmonary fibrosis, chronic obstructive pulmonary disease, secondary pulmonary fibrosis, and pneumoconiosis, accounting for 37.6%, 19.6%, 11.7%, and 11.6%, respectively. Additionally, retransplantation, bronchiectasis, bronchiolitis obliterans, pulmonary hypertension, and lymphangioleiomyomatosis accounted for 4.1%, 3.4%, 2.8%, 1.2%, and 0.3%, respectively (Figure 7–5). Among the cases of idiopathic pulmonary fibrosis, chronic obstructive pulmonary disease, secondary pulmonary fibrosis, and pneumoconiosis, the proportions of bilateral lung transplantation were 57.9%, 61.9%, 70.9%, and 37.6%, respectively.

Chapter 7 Lung Transplantation in China

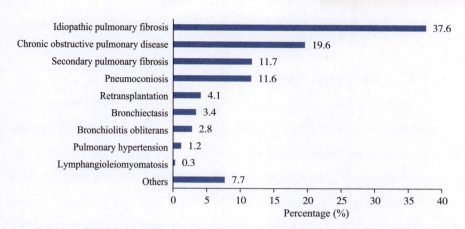

Figure 7-5 Distribution of primary diseases of adult lung transplant recipients in 2023

In 2023, the primary diseases of pediatric lung transplant recipients in China were mainly bronchiolitis obliterans (13 cases), followed by cystic fibrosis (3 cases), pulmonary arteriovenous fistula (2 cases), primary pulmonary hypertension (2 cases), secondary pulmonary fibrosis (1 case), and secondary pulmonary hypertension (1 case) (Figure 7–6).

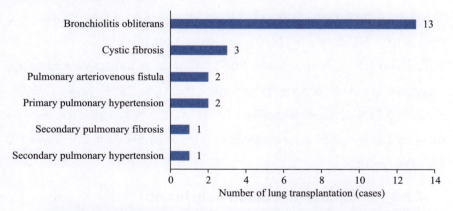

Figure 7-6 Distribution of primary diseases in pediatric lung transplant recipients in China in 2023

7.3 Quality and safety analysis of lung transplantation

7.3.1 Operation methods

In 2023, among adult lung transplantation in China, single lung transplantations and bilateral lung transplantations accounted for 38.5% and 61.3% respectively, while heart–lung combined transplantations accounted for 0.2%. Emergency lung transplantations accounted for 14.2%, and the proportion of surgeries using ECMO was 79.7%. All pediatric lung transplantations were bilateral lung transplantations. Emergency lung transplantations accounted for 13.6%, and the proportion of surgeries using ECMO was 77.3%.

7.3.2 Cold ischemia time

In 2023, the median (interquartile range) cold ischemia times for single and bilateral lung transplantations in China were 6.0 (4.0–7.1) hours and 8.0 (7.0–9.5) hours, respectively. For single lung transplantations, the proportions of cold ischemia times < 2 hours, 2 to < 4 hours, 4 to < 6 hours, 6 to < 8 hours, 8 to < 10 hours, and ⩾ 10 hours were 1.5%, 16.2%, 27.2%, 42.0%, 12.5%, and 0.6%, respectively. For bilateral lung transplantations, the proportions in the corresponding intervals were 0.4%, 3.0%, 12.4%, 26.6%, 35.7%, and 21.9%, respectively (Figure 7–7). In 2023, the median (interquartile range) cold ischemia time for pediatric lung transplantations in China was 8.0 (7.5–9.0) hours.

7.3.3 Intra-operative blood transfusion

The median (interquartile range) intraoperative blood transfusion volume for adult recipients was 800.0 (0.0–1 600.0) mL, with proportions of < 500 mL, 500 to < 1 000 mL, 1 000 to < 1 500 mL, 1 500 to < 2 000 mL and ⩾ 2 000 mL being 39.7%, 17.3%, 14.8%, 9.5%, and 18.7%, respectively. The median (interquartile range) intraoperative blood transfusion volume for pediatric recipients was 650.0 (312.5–2 015.0) mL.

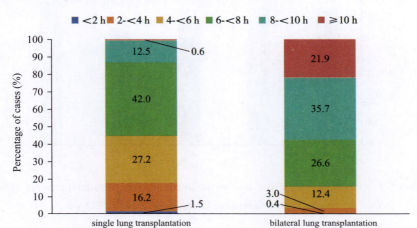

Figure 7-7　Cold ischemia time for single and bilateral lung transplantations in China in 2023

7.3.4　Perioperative complications

In 2023, the incidence rates of graft dysfunction, infection, acute rejection, and tracheal anastomotic lesions before discharge after lung transplantation in China were 15.7%, 66.6%, 3.3%, and 8.8%, respectively. The incidence rates of graft dysfunction from 2019 to 2023 before discharge are shown in Figure 7–8, infection rates are shown in Figure 7–9, acute rejection rates are shown in Figure 7–10, and tracheal anastomotic lesions rates are shown in Figure 7–11.

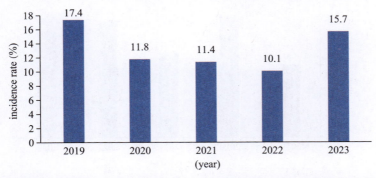

Figure 7-8　Incidence rate of post-operative graft dysfunction before hospital discharge in lung transplant recipients in China from 2019 to 2023

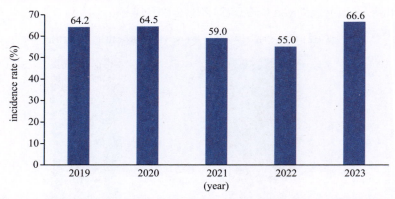

Figure 7-9   Incidence rate of post-operative infection before hospital discharge in lung transplant recipients in China from 2019 to 2023

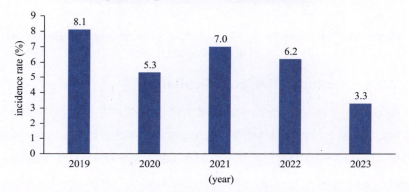

Figure 7-10   Incidence rate of post-operative acute rejection before hospital discharge in lung transplant recipients in China from 2019 to 2023

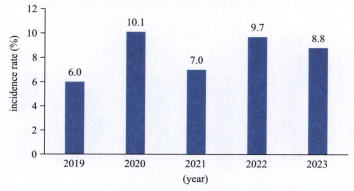

Figure 7-11   Incidence rate of post-operative tracheal anastomotic lesions before hospital discharge in lung transplant recipients in China from 2019 to 2023

7.3.5 Status at discharge

In 2023, the median (interquartile range) ICU stay for adult lung transplantation recipients in China was 144.0 (72.0–336.0) hours, with a median (interquartile range) hospital stay of 32.0 (20.0–49.0) days. For pediatric lung transplantation recipients, the median (interquartile range) ICU stay was 132.0 (87.5–300.5) hours, with a median (interquartile range) hospital stay of 35.0 (30.75–56.0) days. The 30-day survival rate for adult recipients was 83.6%, with the main causes of death within 30 days being multiple organ failure (29.4%), infection (17.5%), hemorrhagic shock (11.1%), and graft dysfunction (6.3%) (Figure 7–12). The causes of death within 30 days for the two pediatric recipients were multiple organ failure and anastomotic complications, respectively.

7.3.6 Post-operation survival

The 30-day, 3-month, 6-month, 1-year, and 3-year post-operation survival rates for recipients of bilateral lung transplantations in China were 82.1%, 70.4%, 63.8%, 58.5%, and 48.4%, respectively, while the corresponding survival rates for recipients of single lung transplantations were 85.9%, 78.2%, 71.4%, 63.6%, and 44.2%, respectively. The short-term survival rates for recipients of single lung transplantations were better than those for recipients of bilateral lung transplantations. The 30-day, 3-month, 6-month and 1-year post-operation survival rates for pediatric lung transplant recipients were 93.7%, 82.0%, 80.4%, and 80.4%, respectively. The postoperative survival rates for recipients with different primary diseases are detailed in Table 7–2.

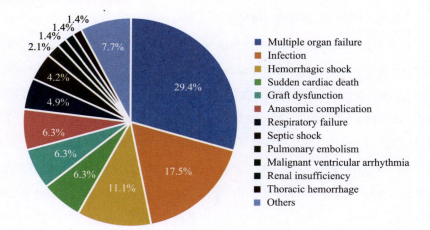

Figure 7-12   Causes of death within 30 days after lung transplantation in adult recipients in China in 2023

Table 7-2   Post-operation survival rate of lung transplant recipients with different characteristics in China

Characteristics	30-day survival rates (%)	3-month survival rates (%)	6-month survival rates (%)	1-year survival rates (%)	3-year survival rates (%)
Type of transplantation					
bilateral lung transplantation	82.1	70.4	63.8	58.5	48.4
single ung transplantation	85.9	78.2	71.4	63.6	44.2
Age of recipients (years)					
< 18	93.7	82.0	80.4	80.4	-
18-34	87.3	78.6	76.3	73.7	65.4
35-49	84.6	77.0	72.2	66.3	59.2
50-59	84.0	76.9	70.4	63.3	48.9
60-64	83.6	71.2	64.1	57.3	41.9
≥ 65	81.8	69.1	60.5	52.7	33.6
Primary disease					
Obliterative bronchiolitis	92.4	78.3	76.7	73.3	63.5
Pneumoconiosis	89.3	83.7	79.6	73.5	64.6
Secondary pulmonary interstitial fibrosis	78.2	65.7	58.9	53.2	37.3

					Continued
Characteristics	30–day survival rates (%)	3–month survival rates (%)	6–month survival rates (%)	1–year survival rates (%)	3–year survival rates (%)
Chronic obstructive pulmonary disease (COPD)	86.9	75.2	67.9	61.2	44.1
Idiopathic pulmonary fibrosis (IPF)	84.2	74.2	66.6	60.1	43.0
Bronchiectasis	82.1	73.4	68.7	60.4	53.4
Pulmonary artery hypertension	74.1	65.5	60.3	54.2	–
Other	76.0	65.7	58.6	53.4	45.1

7.4 Feature and future outlook

7.4.1 The availability of resources and the number of lung transplantations have been consistently increasing, while notable disparities in development exist across various regions

Following the National Health Commission's initiation of the application and certification process for solid organ transplantation qualifications, there has been a yearly increase in the number of hospitals applying for lung transplantation qualifications. Number of hospitals that have successfully passed the review and obtained the qualification has also seen a significant rise.

A comprehensive lung transplantation resource distribution network has been established, encompassing the majority of the country's regions. Nonetheless, regarding the quantity of medical institutions possessing transplantation qualifications in each province, the disproportionate allocation of lung transplantation medical resources persists as a concern. Prominent cities like Guangzhou, Beijing, and Shanghai, along with coastal regions, possess sufficient lung transplantation resources, while resources in the southwestern region are relatively scarce.

From 2015 to 2023, the total number of lung transplants performed nationwide, the number of hospitals actually conducting the surgery, the number of hospitals with more than 10 surgeries, and the number of hospitals with more than 50 surgeries all showed an overall upward trend. However, the issue of uneven regional development in lung transplantation in China remains prominent. In 2023, among the 959 lung transplant surgeries performed nationwide, the top six medical institutions accounted for 69.5% of the total, and only 16 medical institutions performed more than 10 surgeries. Measures should be taken to further promote homogeneous development in this field.

7.4.2 The quality control system for lung transplantation is undergoing continuous improvement, necessitating the ongoing enhancement of transplant quality

In recent years, the National Lung Transplantation Quality Control Center has continuously improved the clinical diagnosis and treatment system for lung transplantation, promoted standardized lung transplantation techniques, intensified publicity efforts for lung transplantation surgeries, and facilitated steady growth in both the number and quality of lung transplants. Through longitudinal monitoring of postoperative complications in transplant recipients over the years, it has been found that the incidence rates of post-transplant airway anastomotic complications and acute rejection after transplantation have declined, while the incidence rates of primary graft failure and perioperative infections have increased. This signifies the necessity for enhanced monitoring and dynamic feedback of quality control indicators, alongside the ongoing development of comprehensive and multifaceted mechanisms for the prevention and management of postoperative complications.

Lung transplantation in China differs significantly from that in developed countries, evident in various aspects such as donor selection, recipient criteria, and postoperative care. In terms of donors, China's organ donation program is still in its nascent phase, and donated lungs pose intricate challenges, including extended mechanical ventilation, aspiration, or infection, necessitating meticulous evaluation to ascertain their viability for safe lung transplantation. In terms of recipients, many lung disease patients in China are elderly and exhibit critical or life-threatening conditions when seeking for lung transplantation. Furthermore, the substantial population may present numerous rare and intricate diseases, requiring the determination of suitable surgical timing and techniques tailored to individual circumstances. When it comes to postoperative management, incidence rates of rejection and infection of lung transplantation in China are significantly higher than that of other solid organ transplantation. Consequently, it is unsuitable to merely replicate international practices, there is a urgent need to summarize previous experiences and formulate a postoperative complication diagnosis and treatment protocol tailored for Chinese patients. The practical challenges encountered in lung transplantation in China have led to a disparity in recipient survival rates relative to international standards. Consequently, developing and advocating for a lung transplantation quality control system tailored to China's specific circumstances is an effective strategy to address these challenges.

7.4.3 Rapid development in pediatric lung transplantation necessitates summarizing relevant experiences and formulating technical documents for the pediatric lung transplantation in China

In recent years, advancements in lung transplantation technology and the accumulation of expertise have enabled several lung transplantation centers in China to perform pediatric lung transplants. Despite the annual volume of pediatric lung transplantations being considerably lower than that of adult operations, from 2019 to 2023, the annual incidence of pediatric lung transplantations in China surged by 36.1%, surpassing the adult lung transplantation growth rate of 23.8%, thereby demonstrating the rapid advancement of pediatric lung transplantation in China over the past five years. Pediatric lung transplants generally show a better prognosis, with a survival rate surpassing 90% within 30 days postoperatively, indicating that the technology of pediatric lung transplantation is progressively advancing and maturing. The immune systems and vital organ functions of children are not fully developed, and their lung growth potential markedly differs from that of adults, resulting in heightened risks and complexities associated with lung transplantation in children compared to adults. They exhibit a higher susceptibility to complications and adverse reactions during surgical procedures and pharmacological interventions. Consequently, there is an imperative necessity to create industry-specific technical guidance documents tailored to China's national context to advance the substantial development of this technology and enhance the long-term outcomes of pediatric lung transplants. In addition, pediatric lung transplantation in China is predominantly centralized in two facilities: Wuxi People's Hospital and the Second Affiliated Hospital of Zhejiang University School of Medicine, highlighting a considerable regional disparity in this technology that requires comprehensive advancement.

Chapter 8 The Development of Technologies and Innovations for Organ Transplantation in China

8.1 Establishment and promotion of key technical system for split liver transplantation

Split liver transplantation is an effective surgical technique that can alleviate donor organ shortage and expand donor organ pool. Despite the fact that liver transplantation in China has been developed for over 40 years, the promotion of split liver transplantation has been slow due to limitations in donor liver availability. Following the comprehensive implementation of donation after citizen death (DCD) in 2015, the proportion of split liver transplantation in China's total liver transplantation remained only 1.25% in 2016, indicating an urgent need to improve and standardize the key technical system for split liver transplantation.

To adapt to the current landscape of solid organ transplantation in China and promote technological innovation, the department of hepatic surgery and liver transplantation center of the Third Affiliated Hospital of Sun Yat-sen University has been conducting split liver transplantation using deceased donor liver since July 2014, with nearly a decade of practice and advancement in this field. To date, we have completed over 200 cases of split liver transplantation and have assisted and guided numerous domestic institutions in carrying out this procedure. We have performed the first complete left and right split liver transplantation with low-age pediatric donor liver (6 years and 4 months old) in China and the world's oldest recipient (82 years old) split liver transplantation, gradually establishing a key technical system for split liver transplantation that can be widely promoted (Figures 8-1 to 8-4).

First, we established the assessment system for split liver grafts, proposing evaluation criteria for splittable liver grafts that include donor age, graft steatosis, graft vascular assessment, donor serum sodium levels, as well as liver ultrasound contrast assessment. The surgical technical workflow for graft segmentation, matching, and reconstruction was also perfected, encompassing the principles of vascular and biliary segmentation and the standards for vascular and biliary reconstruction in both classical and left-right liver splitting. Additionally, corresponding technical solutions were proposed for donor-recipient matching strategies, perioperative management, complication prevention, and long-term follow-up management in split liver transplantation. Furthermore, we have conducted systematic research on split liver graft preservation and post-transplantation regeneration.

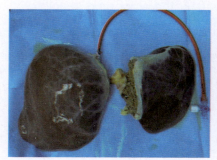

Figure 8-1 Classical isolated split liver transplantation

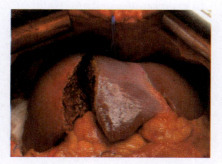

Figure 8-2 In vivo complete split liver transplantation of left and right half liver

Chapter 8 The Development of Technologies and
Innovations for Organ Transplantation in China

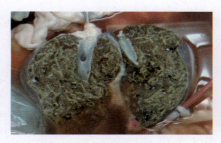 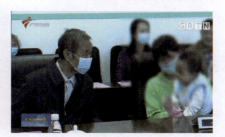

Figure 8-3 Complete left and right splitliver transplantation with splitmiddle hepatic vein

Figure 8-4 In October 2021, the world's oldest recipient (82 year sold) completed split liver transplantation and has been healthy for nearly three years since the surgery

Based on the theoretical and practical advancement of split liver transplantation, active clinical and basic research has been conducted, more than 60 related research articles have been published, including over 30 SCI papers in authoritative journals such as *Hepatology*, *Journal of Hepatology*, and *American Journal of Transplantation*. With the support and participation of colleagues nationwide, we led the publication of the first domestic *Expert Consensus on Split Liver Transplantation* in 2020, as well as the following *Expert Consensus on Donor and Graft Evaluation for Split Liver Transplantation* and the *Chinese Expert Consensus on Vascular Segmentation and Reconstruction in Split Liver Transplantation*. In 2023, we published the first domestic monograph on *Split Liver Transplantation*.

To further promote the development of split liver transplantation, we led the establishment of the first split liver transplantation technology alliance— the South China Split Liver Transplantation Alliance in 2020. Our alliance has consecutively organized four national split liver transplantation academic forums and three national training courses on split liver transplantation, facilitating the application and development of split liver transplantation in China. Through the collective efforts of our colleagues, by 2022, the proportion of split liver transplantation in China had exceeded 8%, and the proportion of split liver grafts used in pediatric liver transplantation had increased from 8% in 2017 to 18.8%. Split liver transplantation has become an imperative part of liver transplantation in China and an outstanding manifestation of independent innovation of liver transplantation in China.

8.2 The AGH score is a predictor of disease-free survival and targeted therapy efficacy after liver transplantation in patients with hepatocellular carcinoma

Technical introduction: Recurrence and metastasis are the most important factors affecting the long-term survival of hepatocellular carcinoma (HCC) after liver transplantation (LT). However, there is a lack of effective ways to stratify the risk of recurrence and metastasis and to identify people who benefit from adjuvant targeted therapy. The present study aimed to establish a new scoring system by screening the parameters related to recurrence and metastasis by Cox regression model to predict HCC recurrence of HCC patients after LT among the Chinese population, and to evaluate whether these patients are suitable for adjuvant targeted therapy.

Technical route: Clinical data of HCC patients who underwent LT from March 2015 to June 2019 were retrospectively collected and analyzed. Results: A total of 201 patients were included in the study. Univariate analysis demonstrated that nine factors were significant predictors of tumor recurrence after LT. These factors included GGT > 96 U/L, AFP > 200 μg/L, total tumor size > 8 cm, largest tumor size > 5 cm, the presence of cancer embolus, the poorer AJCC 8th staging, exceeding the Hangzhou criteria, the Milan criteria and the UCSF criteria. The multivariate Cox analysis suggested that preoperative fetoprotein (AFP), glutamyl transferase (GGT), and beyond Hangzhou criteria were independent risk factors for poor disease-free survival

(DFS) in patients with HCC who underwent LT. We established an AFP-GGT-Hangzhou (AGH) scoring system based on these factors, and divided cases into high-, moderate-, and low-risk groups (Table 8-1). The difference in overall survival (OS) and disease-free survival (DFS) rate among the three groups was significant ($P < 0.05$) (Figure 8-5). The efficacy of the AGH scoring system to predict DFS was better than that of the Hangzhou criteria, UCSF criteria, Milan criteria, and TNM stage (Figure 8-6). Only in the high-risk group, we found that lenvatinib significantly improved prognosis compared with that of the control group ($P < 0.05$) (Figure 8-7).

Table 8-1　AGH score construction

Variables	AGH score
AFP	
≤ 200 μg/L	1
> 200 μg/L	2
GGT	
≤ 96 U/L	1
> 96 U/L	2
Meeting Hangzhou criteria	
Yes	1
No	2
Risk of recurrence	AGH score
Low	3
Moderate	4
High	5-6

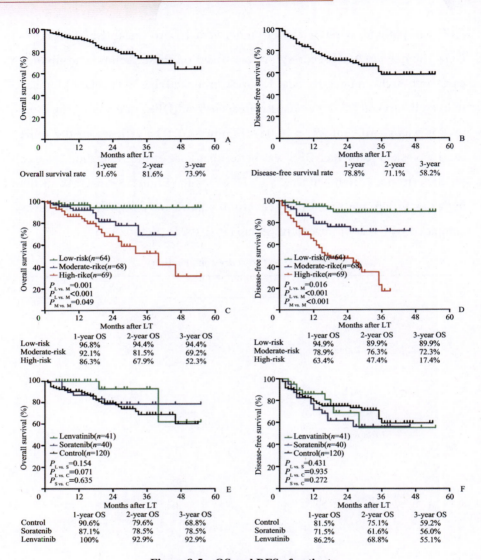

Figure 8-5　OS and DFS of patients

A: Kaplan-Meier OS curve of the whole cohort; B: Kaplan-Meier DFS curve of the whole cohort; C: Kaplan-Meier OS curves among the low-, moderate- and high-risk groups; D: Kaplan-Meier DFS curves among the low-, moderate- and high-risk groups; E: Kaplan-Meier OS curves among the lenvatinib, sorafenib and control groups; F: Kaplan-Meier DFS curves among the lenvatinib, sorafenib and control groups. OS: overall survival; DFS: disease-free survival.

Chapter 8 The Development of Technologies and Innovations for Organ Transplantation in China

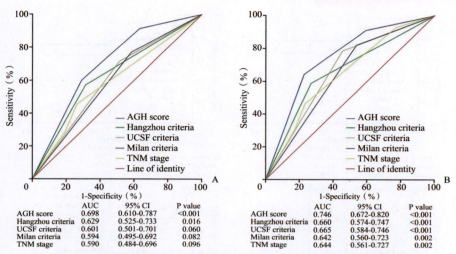

Figure 8-6   Comparison of ROC among Hangzhou, Milan, UCSF criteria, TNM and AGH score

A: The OS of HCC patients who underwent LT; B: The DFS of HCC patients who underwent LT. ROC: receiver operating characteristic; HCC: hepatocellular carcinoma; OS: overall survival; DFS: disease-free survival.

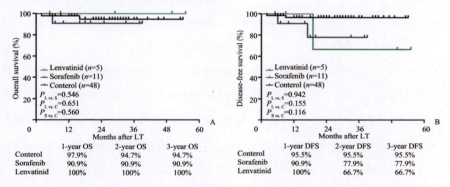

Figure 8-7   Comparison of OS and DFS rates among three groups of patients

A: Kaplan-Meier OS curves among the lenvatinib, sorafenib and control groups in low-risk population; B: Kaplan-Meier DFS curves among the lenvatinib, sorafenib and control groups in low-risk population; C: Kaplan-Meier OS curves among the lenvatinib, sorafenib and control groups in moderate-risk population; D: Kaplan-Meier DFS curves among the lenvatinib, sorafenib and control groups in moderate-risk population; E: Kaplan-Meier OS curves among the lenvatinib, sorafenib and control groups in high-risk population; F: Kaplan-Meier DFS curves among the lenvatinib, sorafenib and control groups in high-risk population. OS: overall survival; DFS: disease-free survival.

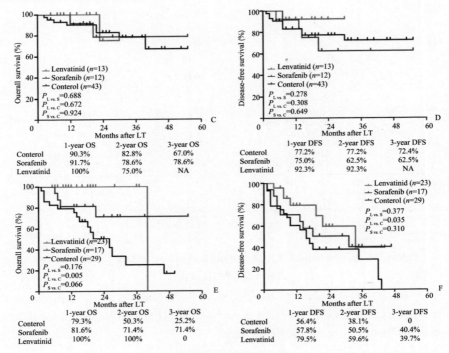

Figure 8-7 Continued

Prospects: AGH scoring system is a convenient and efficient scoring tool for risk stratification of liver cancer recurrence and metastasis based on liver transplantation in Chinese population. For the first time, it introduces the evaluation of the efficacy of targeted drugs to prevent recurrence and metastasis after liver cancer transplantation, which will have high potential for application and promotion under the condition of multi-center verification.

8.3 A novel stratification integrating dual biomarkers in liver transplantation for hepatocellular carcinoma

Liver transplantation (LT) is the most effective treatment for unresectable hepatocellular carcinoma (HCC). Expanding the beneficiary population of LT, reducing tumor recurrence and metastasis, and improving long-term survival rates have always been global challenges with much attention. Scientific and rational recipient selection criteria can significantly improve the therapeutic efficacy of LT and maximize the benefits for recipients. Professor Xu Xiao's research team from Zhejiang University, for the first time, incorporated the key HCC biomarkers protein induced by vitamin K absence or antagonist II (PIVKA- II), also known as des-gamma-carboxy prothrombin (DCP), and alpha-fetoprotein (AFP) into the recipient prognostic stratification system, creating a new classification criteria of LT for HCC.

The team collaborated with six major LT centers in China, including Beijing Tsinghua Changgung Hospital affiliated with Tsinghua University and West China Hospital of Sichuan University, and included a total of 522 cases of LT for HCC patients from 2015 to 2020. By incorporating traditional tumor morphological parameters with molecular parameters including AFP and PIVKA-II, a new prognostic stratification criteria (HC&PIVKA-II) was proposed. When compared to conventional LT criteria, HC&PIVKA-II expanded the beneficiaries from LT by 21.6%, and achieved comparable 1-, 3-, 5-year overall survival rate, with 89.4%, 79.9% and 78.7%, respectively (Figure 8-8).

This study was published in the international surgical authority journal *International Journal of Surgery*. The results closely address the current clinical bottlenecks in LT for HCC and, based on large medicine data from China, further overcome the limitations of traditional LT criteria, enriching the connotation of the new system of individualized precise therapeutic strategy of LT for HCC. Making Chinese contributions and sharing Chinese insights in the field of oncology transplantation.

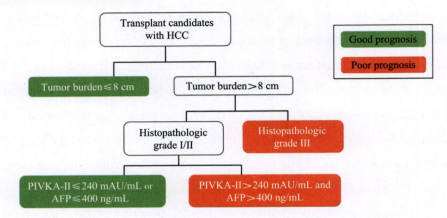

Figure 8-8 The description of the new prognostic stratification criteria based on PIVKA-II

HC&PIVKA-II: (A) tumor burden ⩽ 8 cm; (B) tumor burden > 8 cm, but with histopathologic grade I/II and simultaneously at least 1 eligible tumor markers.

(B1) PIVKA-II ⩽ 240 mAU/mL; (B2) AFP ⩽ 400ng/mL.

8.4 Establishment and application of core technology system for the treatment of multiple organ failure with natural polymer biological liver materials

Liver diseases are major diseases that seriously endanger human health. China is one of the countries with the most serious liver and kidney diseases in the world. The number of new cases of acute and chronic liver failure caused by various causes exceeds 3 million every year. The traditional medical treatment has limited effect, and it is difficult to prevent the deterioration of the disease. Reducing the mortality of liver and kidney failure is an important requirement of the Healthy China strategy. Toxic metabolites produced by hepatic and renal decompensation are common initiating factors for multiple organ failure. Artificial liver can effectively remove toxins from the body and

Chapter 8 The Development of Technologies and Innovations for Organ Transplantation in China

create favorable conditions for liver regeneration and organ function recovery. It is an alternative therapy for patients with liver failure and a bridge for organ transplantation. According to statistics, all kinds of artificial liver treatment costs in the world amount to tens of billions, but the existing artificial liver products are difficult to have both safety and effectiveness, key technical barriers and the cost are high. The development of innovative artificial liver products with excellent comprehensive performance is a breakthrough for the development of this industry.

In order to solve the "bottleneck" problems such as the high mortality rate during the waiting period for transplantation and the poor prognosis effect in patients with severe liver failure (MELD $\geqslant$ 30), after more than 10 years of interdisciplinary cooperation research, the project group has created the core technical system of natural polymer biological liver materials for the treatment of multiple organ failure, and innovated and developed new natural polymer blood purification adsorption materials such as chitin. It can safely, efficiently and accurately adsorb multiple organ failure metabolic toxins such as bilirubin/blood ammonia/creatinine/uric acid/endotoxin, which solves the key technical problem that it is difficult to have both high efficiency and safety of artificial liver adsorption materials. It can be used to improve the internal environment of patients, optimize the quality of donors and organs, and help overcome difficulties in the treatment of multiple organ failure diseases. A novel bioartificial liver reactor was developed and a "trinity" natural polymer bioartificial liver system consisting of chitin–based cell microcarrier, modified hepatocytes and machine perfusion was created, which significantly increased the adherent area of hepatocytes in the reactor, increased cell loading, improved material exchange efficiency, improved cell culture environment, and improved hepatocyte activity. It solves the problem of poor adhesion and viability of hepatocytes in traditional bioartificial liver, and greatly improves the clearance rate of bilirubin and other toxins. The results of clinical trials show that the natural polymer bioartificial liver system can significantly improve the internal environment and liver function of patients, reduce the mortality rate of patients with MELD ⩾ 30 points from 77% to 50%, increase the 1-year survival rate of these patients after liver transplantation to 91% (international reports 58%–65%), reduce the treatment cost by nearly 50%, and benefit the majority of patients (Figure 8-9).

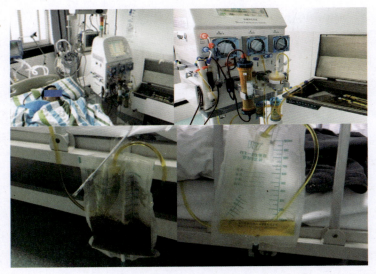

Figure 8-9 Natural polymer bioartificial liver system and its clinical therapeutic effect

The research results have been evaluated by a third party, and the overall results have reached the international leading level. The project has been granted 24 patents (17 invention patents and 7 utility models), and some of them have completed clinical transformation. It has been approved by the Health Commission of Hubei Province as a new medical service pricing and fee item, and has been filed in the National Medical Security Administration. The research platform was approved as Hubei Natural Polymer Bioliver Clinical Medical Research Center; The series of achievements have been supported by more than 20 related scientific research projects, such as the

Chapter 8 The Development of Technologies and Innovations for Organ Transplantation in China

National Natural Science Foundation of China, the Scientific and Technological Innovation Special Project of Hubei Province, and the Natural Science Foundation of Hubei Province. The representative results were published in *Advanced Materials*, *Advanced Functional Material*, *SusMat*, *Carbohydrate Polymers*, *Journal of Materials Chemistry B* and other journals. As the National Quality Control Center for Donateal Organ Procurement, Hubei Province Natural Polymer Bioliver Clinical Medical Research Center, Hubei Hepatobiliary Disease Society, the results have been popularized and applied in more than 20 large tertiary hospitals across the country. The research results were reported in the third issue of *Into Science* program on CCTV-10 Science and Education Channel. The clinical treatment effect was reported by many authoritative media such as People's Daily Online. The achievements won the National Gold Award of the 9th "Creating Youth" China Youth Innovation and Entrepreneurship Competition and the first prize of the Hubei Province Science and Technology Invention Award in 2022.

8.5 Genotype-guided model used for precise anti-rejection therapy after liver transplantation

Background: The success of liver transplantation (LT) depends on the achieving the achievement of an optimal equilibrium between the provision of efficacious immunosuppression and the minimisation of the toxic side effects associated with immunosuppressants. However, with up to 20-fold variation in immunosuppressant doses between patients (0.5-10 mg/d), it is difficult to determine the optimal initial dose of immunosuppressants. Genetic factors account for more than 50% of the metabolic variability. By pharmacogenomics, pharmacokinetics and bioinformatics analysis, we developed a model including major genes (donor CYP3A5 rs776746 and recipient CYP3A5 rs776746), minor genes (recipient SLCO1B1 rs4149015 and recipient CHST10 rs4149015), recipient weight and total bilirubin using lasso regression and accurately differentiated the metabolic type of the receptor tacrolimus with the help of our self-developed fully automated medication intelligence all-in-one machine. Besides, we created a user-friendly web interface for calculating the initial dose after LT according to the panel. In the clinical trial (chiCTR 2100050288), compared to those in experience-based (EB) group, patients in the model-based (MB) group were more likely to achieving the recommended concentration range (75% vs. 40%, $P=0.025$) with a various individual dose as high as 4.2 times (0.023–0.096 mg/kg). Moreover, significantly fewer medication adjustments were required for the MB group than the EB group (2.75 ± 2.01 vs. 6.05 ± 3.35, $P=0.001$), of which the dose can reduce the incidence of acute rejection after LT and the toxicity and adverse reactions of drugs (Figure 8-10).

Progress: The research results have been published in the eClinical-Medicine (IF: 17.033). Based on these findings, a precision drug intelligent integrated system has been developed, and it has obtained a national invention patent (Patent No. ZL 2021 1 1211804.2). Currently, it is being widely promoted and applied in several liver transplant centers.

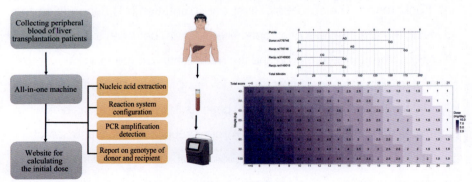

Figure 8-10 Technical route

8.6 Application of Da Vinci robot-assisted laparoscopy in kidney transplantation

Technical introduction: In order to reduce the trauma and incision complications of kidney transplantation, Kunming First People's Hospital combined the special advantages of traditional open surgery and the Da Vinci robot in surgery to perform China's first robotic DD kidney transplantation on February 3rd, 2019. After continuous optimization and improvement of the robotic kidney transplant surgery process, a standard robot-assisted laparoscopic kidney transplant surgery system has been formed. It is currently the center that has performed the largest number of robotic DD kidney transplant surgeries in China, and had the book *Robotic Kidney Transplant Surgery* published by Tsinghua University Press in April, 2023.

Technical route:

1. After trimming the donor kidney, place it in a self-made kidney bag, mark the direction of the transplanted kidney and blood vessels (Figure 8-11A, and 8-11B), and make a self-made single-hole platform (Figure 8-11C).

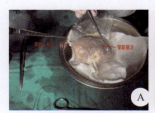 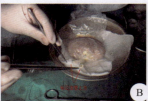 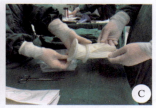

Figure 8-11 Renal repair and labeling

A: The transplanted kidney was put into the kidney bag and the direction was marked; B: Marks the vascular orientation; C: Self-made single-hole platform.

2. Under general anesthesia and intubation, the patient was placed in a supine position with the legs spread apart and the head lowered and the feet higher than 30° (Figure 8-12A).

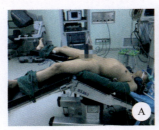 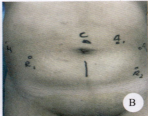 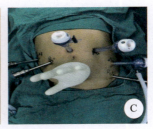

Figure 8-12　Abdominal Trocar position

A: Robotic kidney transplantation position; B: Trocar position Figure; C: Implanted Trocar and self-made channel.

3. Six Trocars were inserted into the abdomen (Figure 8–12B), and the pneumoperitoneum pressure was 13 mmHg. C was the lens Trocar, R1, R2, and R3 were respectively 8 mm Trocars for the robotic arm, and A1 and A2 were 12 mm auxiliary Trocars. A 5–7 cm incision was made in the midline of the abdomen, a self-made single-hole platform was inserted (Figure 8–12C), and the robotic arm was docked (Figure 8–13A).

4. The peritoneum was incised along the lateral abdominal wall, up to about 3 cm above the ileocecal part, and down to below the median umbilical ligament (Figure 8–13B), to establish the renal nest. The external iliac artery and vein were freed extraperitoneally. Place a normal-temperature gauze pad through the single-hole platform (Figure 8–13C), place the transplanted kidney on the gauze pad, and confirm the direction of the transplanted kidney to avoid inversion of the upper and lower poles. The external iliac vein is first blocked, and the recipient's external iliac vein is cut longitudinally according to the diameter of the transplanted renal vein. The vein lumen is repeatedly flushed with heparin saline, and Gore–Tex CV–6 vascular sutures are used to anastomose the renal vein and the external iliac vein end–to–side (Figure 8–13D). Before the venous anastomosis is completed, inject heparin saline to flush the venous lumen again, block the transplanted renal vein, open the vascular blocking clamp of the external iliac vein, and test for leaks. End–to–side

anastomosis between the transplanted renal artery and the recipient's external iliac artery was performed in the same manner (Figure 8-13E). During the operation, ice chips were added to the self-made kidney bag through a single-hole platform to ensure continuous low temperature before the transplanted kidney was opened. The transplanted renal vein and transplanted renal artery were opened in sequence (Figure 8-13F), the reperfusion and ureteral urination of the transplanted kidney were observed, and the transplanted kidney was moved into the renal nest. The posterior bottom wall of the bladder (the side where the transplanted kidney is placed) is incised longitudinally about 2.0cm, and 4-0 absorbable sutures are used to replant the transplanted kidney, ureter, and bladder (Figure 8-13G), and a 5F ureteral stent is left in the ureter. The lateral peritoneum was closed (Figure 8-13H), and the transplanted kidney and transplanted ureter were completely externalized (Figure 8-13I).

Progress and prospects: Currently, Kunming First people's Hospital has completed 121 cases of robotic kidney transplantation, including 98 cases of robotic DD kidney transplantation and 23 cases of robotic LD kidney transplantation. all successfully completed. There were no cases being converted to open surgery. Compared with the open kidney transplantation group, the robotic kidney transplantation group showed no difference in total operation time, arterial anastomosis time, venous anastomosis time, ureteral anastomosis time, blood loss, and creatinine recovery; the hospitalization time and postoperative incision pain were better compared to the open surgery group. Preliminary conclusion: Robot-assisted laparoscopic kidney transplantation is safe and reliable, can achieve the same renal function recovery effect as open surgery, and at the same time speed up the patient's postoperative recovery.

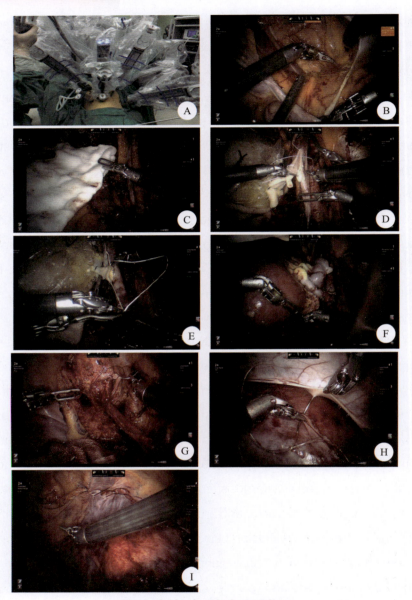

Figure 8-13　Surgical procedure

A: Robot arm docking; B: Cutting the peritoneum; C: Insertion of gauze pad; D: Anastomosis of transplanted renal vein and external iliac vein; E: Anastomosis of the graft artery with the external iliac artery; F: Vascular opening of the transplanted kidney; G: Vesicoureteral anastomosis; H: Suture peritoneum; I: Peritoneal externalization of the transplanted kidney.

8.7 The utilization of an artificial protective external vascular sheath in renal transplantation represents a novel technological advancement aimed at preventing graft artery kinking

The occurrence of a kinked renal artery, which is often observed intraoperatively or in the early postoperative period, represents a rare but serious vascular complication following renal transplantation. In situations where there is a risk of ischemia during surgery, encasing the transplanted renal artery with a protective artificial vascular sheath can effectively ameliorate the kinking status of the anastomotic artery, minimize complications associated with arterial issues, and obviate the need for reoperation.

From January 2019 to June 2022, a total of eight cases of graft artery kinking were identified in the Department of Urology at the First Affiliated Hospital of Soochow University. For rectifying the arterial kink, an innovative technique involving artificial vascular wrapping was employed for transplant renal artery.

All patients underwent an oblique incision to expose the iliac vessels in the lower right abdominal area. Sequential end–to–end arterioarterial anastomosis of the internal iliac artery with 6–0 prolene and side–to–end venovenous anastomosis of the external iliac vein with 5–0 prolene were performed following institutional guidelines. After the graft was placed in the right iliac fossa, a significant kink was observed in the artery (Figure 8–14A). An artificial blood vessel measuring approximately 5 cm in length and 8 mm in diameter (determined by length and diameter of artery) was longitudinally cut (Figure 8–14B) and wrapped around the artery as an external sheath (Figure 8–14C). After discontinuous longitudinal suturing of this artificial blood vessel graft, it was placed again into the right iliac fossa for observation of its blood supply as well as evaluation of renal color and urine ejection.

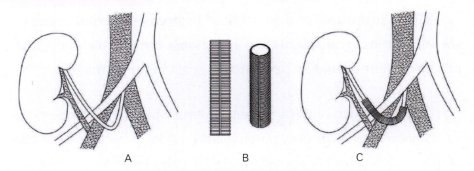

Figure 8-14　Schematic diagram of artificial vascular sheath surgery

All patients, with the exception of one case who experienced delayed graft function (DGF), underwent smooth postoperative recovery. No complications such as acute rejection, fever, wound or pulmonary infections occurred during the perioperative period. On postoperative Day 1, Day 7, and Day 14, color Doppler ultrasound or angiography was performed to assess the blood flow of the graft, and no significant abnormalities were found (Figure 8–15). All patients have been followed up to date without any discomfort in the transplanted kidney area. Regular follow-up color Doppler ultrasound of the transplanted kidney showed no signs of renal artery stenosis. The follow-up pelvic CT scans revealed that the artificial vascular sheath was well-positioned without any leakage or displacement.

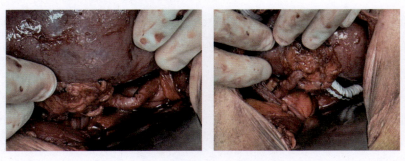

Figure 8-15　Intraoperative transplantation of renal artery torsion and placement of artificial vascular sheath

The artificial ePTFE blood vessel is constructed using expanded polytetrafluoroethylene (ePTFE) and incorporates a support ring made of polytetrafluoroethylene (PTFE) with a blue marked indicator line. It possesses remarkable flexibility, elasticity, compliance, biocompatibility, and the ability to be bent without collapsing. However, there are limited reports on its application as an external sheath for transplanted renal arteries. The external sheath provides exceptional support for the grafted renal artery, resulting in a natural arc in the kinked artery that significantly improves hemodynamics while reducing the risk of compression by surrounding tissues. In this study, eight patients achieved favorable outcomes following arterial wrapping. The strong biocompatibility of the artificial ePTFE vasculature and its anti-infective properties have demonstrated clinical success and may confer reduced susceptibility to infection (Figure 8-16).

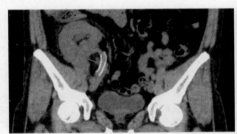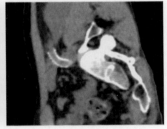

Figure 8-16 Artificial vascular sheath (CT axial and sagittal)

The protective artificial ePTFE external vascular sheath, in summary, effectively rectifies a kinked anastomotic artery, enhances blood supply, and minimizes the risk of long-term stenosis in the transplanted renal artery with exceptional stability, utmost safety, and minimal complications.

8.8 Six-genes edited porcine-rhesus kidney xenotransplantation

A gene-edited porcine-rhesus kidney xenotransplantation was performed on Oct. 27th 2023 by the Department of Urology of the First Hospital affiliated to Air Force Medical University. A porcine donor with 6 gene edits was used in the experiment, with 3 known glycan antigens that were known to cause hyperacute rejection, together with the transgenic expression of 2 complement regulatory proteins and 1 thromboregulatory protein. The researches transplanted the left porcine kidney to the right abdomen of the recipient monkey. The xenograft artery and vein were anastomosed to the recipient's abdominal artery and inferior vena cava in a end-to-side manner, respectively. The xenograft ureter was anastomosed to the bladder using the Lich-Gregoir technique. The recipient's native kidneys were resected simultaneously, so that the xenograft functioned as the life-sustaining kidney, and this mimicked the situation that patient with uremia received kidney transplantation in the clinical setting. Induction therapy included anti-thymocyte globulin, anti-CD20 antibody and complement inhibition. Maintenance immunosuppressive regimens included tacrolimus, mycophenolate mofetil and steroid (Figure 8-17).

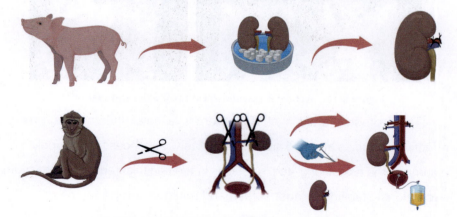

Figure 8-17 Schematic overview of the experiment

The xenograft kidney functioned well the first week after transplantation, with urine output ranged from 585–2 543 mL per day. The serum creatinine level was kept stable, and screening with Doppler ultrasound showed excellent blood perfusion in the xenograft (Figure 8-18). Starting from POD9, the urine output started to decline and serum creatinine level increased. Biopsy of the xenograft showed acute antibody-mediated rejection. Steroid pulse, anti-CD20 antibody and intravenous immunoglobulin were applied but failed to reverse the rejection. Repeated biopsy showed aggravated antibody-mediated rejection. The recipient rhesus was euthanized on POD27.

The current study demonstrated that the gene-edited porcine donor, together with clinical grade immunosuppressive regimens were sufficient to prevent hyperacute rejection and achieved relatively long survival of the xenograft. However, acute antibody-mediated rejection was not prevented, possibly due to the absence of co-stimulation pathway blockage. In future study, we will improve our protocol and try to prolong the survival of porcine-rhesus kidney xenograft, so as to provide knowledge and experience for the clinical application of kidney xenotransplantation.

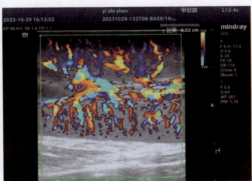

Figure 8-18　Colorful Doppler imaging showed excellent blood perfusion of the xenograft

8.9　The first group of 37 cases of kidney transplantation for infants and young children in China

Compared with long-term dialysis, kidney transplantation can significantly improve the survival rate and quality of life of patients with end-stage renal disease, especially kidney transplantation in young children, which can not only save the lives of children, but also meet the growth and development needs of children. In 1979, Tongji Hospital Affiliated to Tongji Medical College of Huazhong University of Science and Technology implemented the first child kidney transplant in China, receiving adult donor kidney transplantation for children aged 19 months, and the children survived for 10 years. In the following 30 years, the number of infant kidney transplants in China is very small, especially the infant kidney transplantation under 1 year old has been in a blank state. After entering a new era of organ donation in 2015, organ donation after the death of children became possible, which greatly promoted the rapid development of pediatric kidney transplantation. Tongji Hospital Affiliated to Tongji Medical College of Huazhong University of Science and Technology completed the first infant kidney transplantation in China in 2017, accepting kidney donation for 6-month-old children with congenital nephrotic syndrome who died of trauma at 5-monthold. From then to July 31, 2022, Tongji Hospital has implemented a total of 37 cases of kidney transplantation for children <3 years old (accounting for the vast majority in China). Among them, 13 cases (35.1%) of infant kidney transplantation were <1 year old, and 7 cases (18.9%) of infant kidney transplantation were <6 months old. The youngest recipient was only 2 months and 26 days old, weighing 3.2 kg, which was the youngest child kidney transplantation case in the world.

The 37 recipients had a median age of 16 months (range: 2 months, 26 days to 36 months) and a median body weight of 8 kg (range: 3.2 to 14.0 kg). All kidney donors came from organ donation after the death of children. Except for one donor whose age was 10 years old, the age of all the other donors was less than 3 years old, the minimum age was 9 days, and the median age was 7 months (Figure 8-19A). The minimum weight is 2.8 kg and the median weight is 6.0 kg (Figure 8–19B). The most common cases were congenital nephrotic syndrome (13 cases, 41.9%). Intra-abdominal transplantation occurred in 19 cases (51.3%) and intra-iliac fossa transplantation occurred in the remaining 18 cases (48.6%). The 1-year and 2-year survival rates of the grafts were 85.3%, and the 1-year and 2-year survival rates of the recipients were 96.8% (Figure 8–20).

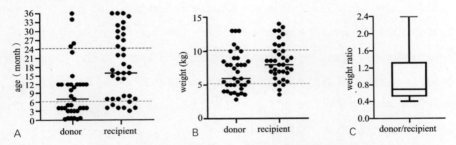

Figure 8-19 Age and weight distribution of kidney transplant donors and recipients

A: Age distribution of donors and recipients; B: Donor and recipient weight distribution; C: Donor/recipient weight ratio; 36 donors were shown in A and B, and 1 10-year-old donor was not shown in the figure.

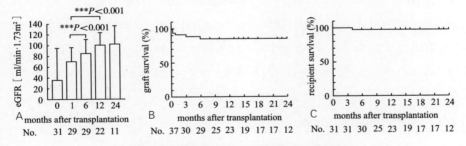

Figure 8-20 Survival of grafts and recipients

A: Estimated glomerular filtration rate (eGFR) changes after kidney transplantation; B: graft survival curve; C: Recipient survival curve.

Although the operation and postoperative management of infant kidney transplantation are extremely difficult, this study still achieved better transplant results compared with the international level. The results indicate that the kidney transplantation of infants can achieve relatively satisfactory clinical results after delicate operation and multi-disciplinary management. The practice of this group of cases provides valuable early experience for young children in China and even in the world to use infant kidney donor for transplantation.

8.10 Ischemia-free heart transplantation

On June 26, 2021, the First Hospital of Sun Yat-sen University to successfully complete the world's first ischemia-free heart transplantation, which resulted in the patient's long-term survival. Prof. Yin Shengli, as one of the main authors, published the article Transplantation of a Beating Heart: A First in Man in *The Lancet Regional Health Western Pacific* in 2022, and participated in the writing and publication of the book *IschemiaFree Organ Transplantation* in 2023, Ischemia-Free Organ Transplantation is Using extracorporeal normothermic mechanical attention support and innovative surgical methods, it realizes that blood flow is not interrupted during the whole process of donor organ acquisition and recipient organ implantation, and the organ is always supplied with blood and oxygen, which fundamentally eliminates the impact of ischemia-reperfusion injury on organ function during organ acquisition and transplantation, and significantly reduces the incidence of complications such as delayed recovery of organ function and acute rejection after organ transplantation.

This book mainly focuses on introducing the history, current status and problems of organ transplantation; explaining the concept of ischemia-free organ transplantation in detail; describing the harm of ischemia-reperfusion injury on transplanted organs;the relationship between ischemia-reperfusion injury and immunity; elaborating ischemia-free organ (liver, kidney, heart) transplantation, including the method of normothermic mechanical perfusion of the liver, kidney, and heart outside of the body; anesthesia management for ischemia-free organ transplantation; and describing the ischemia-free Transplantation of Ischemia-Free Organs: Prospects for Organ Medicine, and nine other chapters on Ischemia-Free Organ Transplantation.

8.11 A novel myocardial biopsy technique after heart transplantation

1. Technical introduction

Heart transplantation is an effective treatment for all types of end-stage heart disease, and rejection remains one of the leading causes of death. Myocardial biopsy is the "gold" standard for diagnosing rejection. The endomyocardial biopsy commonly used in clinical practice is the technique of using catheterized biopsy forceps to clip endocardial myocardial tissues from the right ventricle or the left ventricle through peripheral blood vessels under radiation. Because of the high technical difficulty and the small amount of pathological tissue specimens in a single biopsy, fewer hospitals are able to carry out this technique independently, and the development of this technique is limited.

In 2023, Zhongnan Hospital of Wuhan University adopted a brand-new method of myocardial biopsy, namely the ultrasound-guided percutaneous puncture of the interventricular septum for myocardial biopsy. Now, we summarize the operation of this technique as well as its advantages and disadvantages.

2. Technical route (Figure 8-21 to Figure 8-22)

1) Operation process

(1) According to the preparation of general anesthesia, fasting for 12 hours before surgery, and forbidding drinking for 4-6 hours; Patients need to sign the

informed consent form.

(2) The patient was placed in the left lateral position, the right shoulder pad was 30–40 degrees high. Intravenous general anesthesia was administered through laryngeal mask.

(3) The S5–1 ultrasound probe was protected with a sterile sleeve. After disinfecting and spreading the towel, load the LEAPMED A–type puncture guidance frame (3 530) on the ultrasound probe. After the transthoracic ultrasound has clarified that there are no coronary vessels on the puncture path, determine the route of the needle, and then put the Bard Mission Disposable Core Biopsy Instrument into the 17G card slot of the LEAPMED A–type puncture frame. The puncture needle penetrates the skin, intercostal muscle, pericardium, and apical ventricular wall muscle to the ventricular septum sequentially.

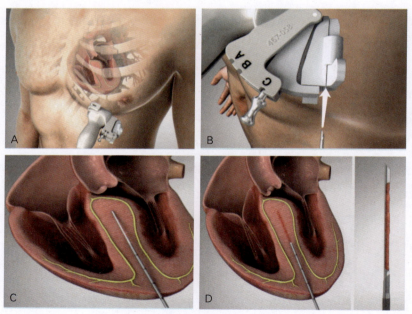

Figure 8-21　Simulation of ultrasound-guided percutaneous intra ventricular septal myocardial biopsy

(4) Remove the slot for the puncture guide and determine by ultrasound that the biopsy needle is located within the ventricular septum, which should be positioned more than 3 mm from the endocardial surfaces of the left and right ventricles, and the tip should be more than 20 mm from the aortic annulus. Activate the biopsy needle and obtain myocardial tissue within the ventricular septum 10 mm × 1 mm at one time.

(5) Withdraw the needle, remove the myocardial tissue from the slot hole of the biopsy needle, and send it to the Department of Pathology for pathological examination.

(6) Ultrasonic real–time observation for 5–10 minutes, to determine the absence of pericardial effusion, the puncture point of local disinfection and bandage, the patient is awake back to the ward.

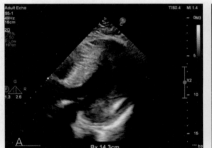 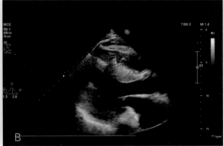

Figure 8-22 Ultrasound-guided percutaneous intra ventricular septal myocardial biopsy

2) Advantages and disadvantages (Table 8-2)

Table 8-2 Advantages and disadvantages

	Advantages	Disadvantages
DSA-guided transcatheter EMB	Local anaesthesia	DSA radiographs; small single sample size; Susceptible to right ventricular injury, pericardial effusion; blind grasping; high cost
Ultrasound-guided transseptal intraventricular MB	Ultrasound guidance; no radiation; visualization; Large sample size at one time; few complications; Short learning curve and low input costs	New technology; general anesthesia; ultrasound collaboration required

3. Stage progress and expected prospects

Zhongnan Hospital of Wuhan University has successfully implemented this technique in 15 cases, all of which were successful, with an average procedure time of 5–10 minutes, pericardial effusion in 1 case (ECMO–assisted patient), and no other complications. The method is simple to operate, learning curve segment, with the characteristics of visualization, repeatable, green and radiation–free, large volume of single biopsy specimen, etc. Compared with the traditional method, it has significant advantages, and it has the potential to be popularized and widely applied in myocardial biopsy after heart transplantation.

8.12 A machine learning based prognostic model for lung transplant patients

In recent years, China has made significant advancements in lung transplantation surgical techniques and perioperative management. However, the survival rate of lung transplant recipients remains suboptimal. Improving the long–term survival and quality of life of recipients is a critical issue of global concern in the field of lung transplantation. Improving the long–term survival and quality of life of recipients is a critical issue in the global lung transplantation field. Developing accurate survival prediction tools is essential for transplant physicians to create individualized management plans, thereby improving recipient prognosis. In this context, Prof. Jingyu Chen and his team, utilizing Chinese lung transplant clinical data, were the first to employ artificial intelligence methods to construct a prognostic model for the continuous survival of lung transplant recipients post–surgery. They also used the random survival forest (RSF) machine learning algorithm to develop and validate a prognostic model for predicting the overall survival of lung transplant recipients. This study found that the RSF model demonstrated strong predictive performance for the survival outcomes of lung transplant recipients, with an integrated area under the curve (iAUC) value of 0.879. Additionally, under the same modeling conditions, the predictive performance of the RSF model significantly surpasses that of the traditional Cox regression model. It is worth noting that according to the optimal threshold predicted by the RSF model, lung transplant recipients can be stratified into prognoses. The overall survival of the low-risk group and the high-risk group was significantly different, with an average overall survival of 52.9 months and 14.8 months, respectively. This result demonstrates the significant potential of artificial intelligence methods in the field of lung transplantation, providing a crucial preliminary foundation for future research and advancing the clinical application of these techniques. This artificial intelligence model can offer practical and reliable guidance for transplant physicians in their management decisions, ultimately enhancing the long-term survival and quality of life of lung transplant recipients.

On May 5, 2023, the study was published in *JAMA Network Open* (*impact facter: 13.88, Zone 1,* Chinese Academy of Sciences), a journal affiliated with the American Medical Association (JAMA). This marks the first time that clinical lung transplant data from China has been accepted by a leading international journal. This achievement is of significant importance for the advancement of clinical medicine in the field of lung transplantation within our country. It also offers valuable insights and guidance for future clinical practices in lung transplantation nationally. Due to historical reasons, some organizations and individuals in the international community still hold prejudices against China's organ transplantation efforts. The acceptance of Jingyu Chen team's research results by a JAMA journal indicates that China's lung transplantation efforts are gradually gaining international recognition. This achievement demonstrates that the level of clinical research in lung transplantation within

China has increasingly aligned with international standards. It significantly advances China's external exchanges and cooperation in the field, marking a groundbreaking step in elevating China's lung transplantation efforts to a prominent position on the global stage.

8.13 Robot-assisted lung transplantation

1. Technical introduction

Currently, most lung transplant procedures, including double and single lung transplants, are performed through open incisions such as Clamshell or standard posterolateral incisions. However, these extremely invasive approaches may contribute to early post-operative pain, delay wound healing, and cause chronic post-thoracotomy neuralgia, which can affect patient's quality of life. Compared to traditional lung transplant surgery, robot-assisted minimally invasive lung transplantation offers several advantages:

(1) Minimally invasive surgical incisions facilitate accelerated postoperative recovery. Minimally invasive lung transplant surgery features smaller incisions, resulting in reduced trauma, better preservation of respiratory muscle function, lighter postoperative pain, and enhanced postoperative respiratory function and cough strength, thus expediting recovery.

(2) Precise suturing reduces procedural complexity. The crux of lung transplant surgery lies in the precise anastomosis of the bronchus, pulmonary artery, and left atrial cuff. The greatest advantage of the da Vinci robotic surgical system lies in its capability to perform intricate operations such as suturing in confined spaces. With flexible mechanical arms enabling 360° rotation, the system facilitates precise, rapid, and comprehensive suturing without blind spots.

(3) Effective hemostasis enhances safety. Robot-assisted minimally

invasive lung transplant surgery allows for more precise dissection of adhesions, thorough examination of each bleeding point, and accurate, adequate hemostasis.

2. Technical route

Qingdao University Affiliated Hospital made full use of the advantages of the da Vinci robot, such as the three-dimensional high-definition vision and flexible rotating wrist equipment, which allowed us to perform difficult dissections, reliable hemostasis, and precise anastomosis. Using robot-assisted lung transplantation, the anastomoses (including of the bronchus, pulmonary artery, and left atrial cuff) were performed using a half-continuous suture method. All procedures, including suturing and knot tying, were performed by robotic instruments. Additionally, to deal with unexpected intra-operative conditions, the assistant at the operating table requires a high level of training and should be able to independently perform minimally invasive lung surgery (Figure 8-23).

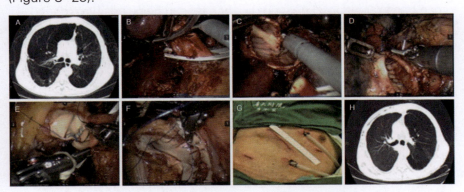

Figure 8-23 Minimally invasive lung surgery

A: Pre-operative chest computed tomography of the recipient; B: The pulmonary artery was cut by robotic scissors; C: The right main bronchus was cut by robotic scissors; D: End-to-end half-continuous anastomosis for the bronchus; E: Anastomosis for the pulmonary artery; F: Anastomosis for the left atrium; G: The skin incision was closed with an intradermal suture; H: Post-operative chest computed tomography of the recipient.

In April 2022, the team led by Dr. Wenjie Jiao from the Department of Thoracic Surgery at the Affiliated Hospital of Qingdao University successfully performed Asia's first robot-assisted single lung transplant, with a follow-up period of 27 months.

In February 2023, the world's first robot-assisted lung transplantation article was published (*Chinese Medical Journal*, Zone 1 of Science Citation Index, impact factor: 7.5).

8.14 Application of donor-derived cell-free DNA in diagnosing rejection after lung transplantation

Donor-derived cell-free DNA (dd-cfDNA) refers to the free DNA from apoptotic or necrotic donor cells in the circulating body fluids of organ transplant recipients, carrying cellular information from the donor tissue. In recent years, dd-cfDNA has become a research hotspot in the field of solid organ transplantation. Published data and research findings have deepened the understanding of dd-cfDNA in transplant-related injuries, especially acute rejection. Dd-cfDNA is expected to become a promising non-invasive biomarker for the future detection of rejection in lung transplantation. However, there is a lack of relevant research in the field of lung transplantation in China.

The lung transplant team at the First Affiliated Hospital of Guangzhou Medical University has pioneered two retrospective clinical studies related to dd-cfDNA in lung transplant recipients in China. The first study included 170 lung transplant recipients, which were divided into infection, acute rejection, chronic lung allograft dysfunction (CLAD), and stable groups. It compared the plasma dd-cfDNA levels among the four groups and found that the acute rejection and CLAD groups had significantly higher dd-cfDNA levels than the infection and stable groups ($P<0.05$) (Figure 8-24A). Using 1.17%

as the threshold, the sensitivity and specificity of dd–cfDNA in diagnosing acute rejection were 89.19% and 86.47%, respectively. Additionally, there was a significant difference in dd–cfDNA levels before and after treatment, with levels significantly decreasing after treatment (Figures 8–24B, Figures 8–24C). This study is the first in China to explore the application of dd–cfDNA in diagnosing lung transplant recipients, laying the foundation for using dd–cfDNA for non–invasive monitoring of lung transplant recipient conditions. The second study, building on the first, was the first to correlate dd–cfDNA results with metagenomic next–generation sequencing (mNGS) results of bronchoalveolar lavage fluid (BALF). This study included 188 lung transplant recipients, divided into rejection, infection, and stable groups. The study found that in lung transplant recipients, plasma dd–cfDNA levels continuously decreased over time, stabilizing approximately one month post–operation if no rejection occurred (Figure 8–24D). In the infection group, dd–cfDNA levels increased with cytomegalovirus infection but did not significantly change with bacterial or fungal infections. The combination of dd–cfDNA and mNGS results significantly improved the diagnostic efficiency of dd–cfDNA for rejection. The positive predictive value and negative predictive value for diagnosing rejection were 88.7% and 99.2%, respectively, when dd–cfDNA levels were elevated, and mNGS results were negative (Figure 8–24E). In conclusion, we have, for the first time, detected dd–cfDNA levels in the Chinese lung transplant population, providing baseline data for dd–cfDNA in Chinese lung transplant recipients.

In summary, this study is the first research on dd–cfDNA in Chinese lung transplant recipients, providing baseline data for dd–cfDNA in this population. It initially elucidates the application of dd–cfDNA in diagnosing post–lung transplantation complications, laying the foundation for using dd–cfDNA as a non–invasive method to monitor post–lung transplantation complications.

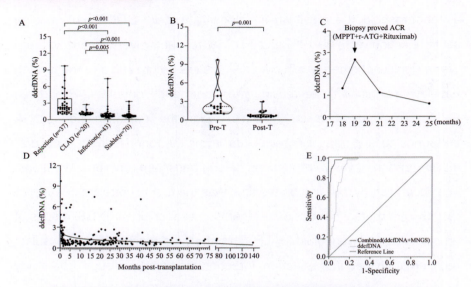

Figure 8-24 The application of dd-cfDNA in lung transplant recipients

A: Plasma dd–cfDNA levels among different groups; B: Plasma dd–cfDNA levels significantly decrease after treatment; C: In lung tissue pathology–confirmed grade 3 rejection, dd–cfDNA levels significantly increase before treatment and gradually decrease with treatment improvement; D: In lung transplant recipients, plasma dd–cfDNA levels gradually decrease over time, reaching a steady state approximately one month post–operation; E: Combining dd–cfDNA with mNGS results can improve the sensitivity and specificity of dd–cfDNA in diagnosing rejection.